BACK PAIN REHABILITATION

Back Pain Rehabilitation

Edited by

Brian P. D'Orazio, PT, MS

Orthopedic and Sports Physical Therapy Associates, Inc.
Fredericksburg, Virginia

With 14 Contributing Authors

Andover Medical Publishers

Boston London Oxford Singapore Sydney Toronto Wellington

Andover Medical Publishers is an imprint of Butterworth–Heinemann.

Copyright © 1993 by Butterworth–Heinemann

ℛ A member of the Reed Elsevier group
All rights reserved.

Every effort has been made to ensure that the drug dosage schedules within this text are accurate and conform to standards accepted at time of publication. However, as treatment recommendations vary in the light of continuing research and clinical experience, the reader is advised to verify drug dosage schedules herein with information found on product information sheets. This is especially true in cases of new or infrequently used drugs.

∞ Recognizing the importance of preserving what has been written, it is the policy of Butterworth–Heinemann to have the books it publishes printed on acid-free paper, and we exert our best efforts to that end.

Library of Congress Cataloging-in-Publication Data

Back pain rehabilitation / edited by Brian D'Orazio ; with 14
   contributing authors.
     p.   cm.
   Includes bibliographical references and index.
   ISBN 1-56372-029-9 (alk. paper)
   1. Backache—Patients—Rehabilitation.   2. Backache—Treatment.
   3. Backache—Psychological aspects.   I. D'Orazio, Brian.
   [DNLM: 1. Low Back Pain—rehabilitation.   WE 755 B1263 1993]
   RD771.B217B335   1993
   617.5'6403—dc20
   DNLM/DLC
   for Library of Congress   93-11017
                                            CIP

British Cataloging-in-Publication Data.

A catalogue record for this book is available from the British Library.

Butterworth–Heinemann
313 Washington Street
Newton, MA 02158–1626

10 9 8 7 6 5 4 3 2

Printed in the United States of America

Contents

Contributing Authors

Gunnar B. J. Andersson, MD, PhD
Department of Orthopedic Surgery
Rush-Presbyterian-St. Luke's Medical Center
Chicago, Illinois

Ronald C. Childs, MD
Department of Orthopedic Surgery
Rush-Presbyterian-St. Luke's Medical Center
Chicago, Illinois

Don Darling, MS, PT
Physical Therapy Orthopaedic Specialists, Inc.
Minneapolis, Minnesota

Brian P. D'Orazio, PT, MS
Orthopedic and Sports Physical Therapy Associates, Inc.
Fredericksburg, Virginia

Barbara Danahy Ehman, PT
Orthopedic and Sports Physical Therapy Associates, Inc.
Fredericksburg, Virginia

Susan J. Isernhagen, PT, PhD
Isernhagen and Associates, Inc.
Isernhagen Work Systems
Duluth, Minnesota

Robert B. King, PT
Vice President
Practice Development Division
Healthfocus
Lakewood, Colorado

Paul L. Lysher, PT, ATC
Orthopedic and Sports Physical Therapy Associates, Inc.
Fredericksburg, Virginia

Philip W. Meilman, PhD
Research Associate Professor
Department of Psychology
Director, Counseling Center
College of William & Mary
Williamsburg, Virginia

Mohamad Parnianpour, PhD
Assistant Professor
Department of Industrial and Systems Engineering
Associate Director
Biodynamics Laboratory
The Ohio State University
Columbus, Ohio

Serge H. Roy, ScD, PT
Research Assistant Professor
Neuromuscular Research Center
Boston University
Senior Research Associate
Loss Prevention
Liberty Mutual Insurance Company
Boston, Massachusetts

Jackson C. Tan, PhD, MD, PT
Adjunct Assistant Professor
Program of Ergonomics & Biomechanics
New York University
Coordinator, Muscle Laboratory
Occupational Industrial and Orthopaedic Center
Hospital for Joint Diseases
New York, New York

Kent E. Timm, PhD, PT, SCS, OCS, ATC, FACSM
Instructor
Physical Therapy Department
University of Michigan
Flint, Michigan
Sports/Industrial Medicine Consultant
St. Luke's Health Care Association
St. Luke's Hospital
Saginaw, Michigan

Timothy C. Toomey, PhD
Associate Professor
Department of Psychiatry
University of North Carolina Medical School
Chapel Hill, North Carolina

Preface

This text presents back pain rehabilitation as a multidimensional process leading to measurable, functional outcomes. Each chapter is part of an integrated whole, systematically examining this complex process as an amalgam of treatment, exercise, psychosocial assessment, patient management, and measurement of functional impairment. Most important, *Back Pain Rehabilitation* presents usable clinical skills from the disciplines of psychology, engineering, occupational medicine, manual therapy, medicine, and physical therapy.

The text is divided into three parts: Rehabilitation, Assessment and Management Strategies, and Functional Considerations. None of the parts is exhaustive in scope. This is purposeful both to prevent the reader from becoming mired in technique and to promote the main purpose of the text, an integration of topics. Gregory Grieve's preface to *Modern Manual Therapy of the Vertebral Column* (Churchill Livingstone, 1986) notes "technique is not of prime importance, since technique springs most naturally from the fullest grasp of the nature of the musculo-skeletal problem. More arduous than learning the various ways to push this or tweak and pull that is the task of educating oneself in understanding the problem." With this in mind, the parts are not exclusively devoted to the discussion of technique, but rather emphasize approaches to patient care. They represent information that compiles the best research available with the most current clinical thinking supported by reasonable empirical evidence.

Part I, Rehabilitation, begins by examining many of the techniques and philosophies used by renowned clinicians around the world. Over the past two decades, clinicians have engaged in theoretical debates over which techniques are most effective. The obvious commonality in these discussions is that everyone feels their treatment method is effective. If the premise is accepted that given treatments are effective, until research validates technique, we must draw from the commonalities of treatments and integrate them into a mature philosophy that emphasizes approach more than technique.

Much as treatment approaches and techniques are part of the clinician's rehabilitation armamentarium, so too is the ability to prescribe exercise for low back pain (LBP). Exercise as a treatment for LBP has sound statistical support in the research literature, demonstrating that properly prescribed exercise limits disability associated with LBP and can reduce time lost from work. When surgical intervention is required, many of the same principles for exercise prescription can be followed, but with more attention paid to soft tissue healing times. Despite the common use of postoperative rehabilitation, no research supports specific approaches. Consequently, chapter 3, Rehabilitation after Back Surgery, provides guiding principles for LBP rehabilitation based on known tissue healing times and clinical experience.

Part II, Assessment and Management Strategies, examines psychosocial assessment and its relationship to selected management strategies. The complex interrelationships between the body and the mind make it clear why LBP treatment often fails. Psychosocial events can produce barriers to a patient's recovery. One of the greatest clinical challenges is to recognize barriers to recovery and make sure that the clinician is not one of those barriers. The clinician plays a substantial role in simply ameliorating fears and anxieties. For many patients, specific management strategies lead to successful outcomes, even in a chronic pain population. Misguided approaches can propel a patient into chronic pain, leading to protracted and irrevocable disability. A failure in treatment is often not the result of improper technique, but rather a signal that a mental health professional should be consulted. Specific examples of how to work with a patient behaviorally are presented in this section. We hope that the reader will learn techniques for behavior modification and warning signs for patients who are in danger of failing or placing themselves in danger because of depression.

Part III, Functional Considerations, examines functional assessments and isolated factors that contribute to impairment. Impairment is increasingly defined as a separate entity from disability. A great clinical challenge is to define the difference objectively. Many tools are available that, if used appropriately, can help in this process. Ultimately, we may have to use our best clinical judgment, but at least we should be able to define where our knowledge ends and where the art of clinical practice takes over. This part truly is a combination of clinical science and clinical art. One goal of this text is to define the line between these two entities. As research advances, it is everyone's hope that treatment techniques will be validated and performance can be more accurately measured. By considering all the variables currently known, including lumbar fatigue, it is my hope that this part of the text will allow the clinician to make informed choices.

This will be the decade that allows clinicians to view LBP treatment as a process, leading to more fulfilling clinical interactions with patients. Mature debates will take place about relative efficacy of approaches and the approach itself. While techniques and skills are important, they are, after all, a means to an end. As Grieve again notes in his preface, "Many recent advances in basic knowledge and alternative ways of thinking about old problems, have already made our yesterdays seem centuries ago, yet we need to recognize sterile propaganda and plain advertisement. Novelty is not progress." Indeed, new approaches are not necessarily good approaches. Clinicians must maintain objectivity and be familiar with the many brilliant works of research published over the past 20 years. It is my hope that the reader will enjoy the challenge of integrating this perspective of LBP rehabilitation into clinical practice.

The experience of putting together this text has been personally cathartic. It has given me the opportunity to speak with some of the best in the field and share concerns, ideas, and frustrations on a variety of topics. Each author enthusiastically embraced the ideas put forth in the proposal for this text and each was eager to contribute. Implicit in their excitement is the hope that information in this text may touch the lives of many clinicians and ultimately their patients. In the final analysis, our main purpose is to help as best we can with the knowledge and gifts given to each of us.

Brian P. D'Orazio

Acknowledgments

Much energy and excitement goes into the publication of a text. In the two and a half years that it took to complete this work, individuals behind the scenes have been extremely helpful in guiding my ideas about the presentation of this material. It has been a most enjoyable experience. I would like to thank each contributor to this text. It has truly been a pleasure to exchange ideas and information with such gifted individuals. They have all given of their time unselfishly and have shared a wealth of knowledge that kept me excited about this project throughout its course. I would also like to thank many of the individuals who have helped focus my ideas, especially Rebecca Guy for her help in reading some of the material for this text and giving appropriate literary criticism. Robert King was gracious enough to offer suggestions for my chapter and Cynthia Starling has been helpful in organizing the information. Much appreciation is extended to Patricia Retter, Stephanie Harlow, and Tina Ellison for their contributions in manuscript preparation and much leg work.

Reserving an editor's right, this text is compassionately dedicated to our patients with low back pain. I pray that the contributions in this text will serve to advance low back pain treatment.

BPD

□ □ □
□ □ □
□ □ □

Introduction

Most low back pain articles, books, research, prefaces, etc., begin by examining the ubiquity of low back pain (LBP) and its fiscal consequences. Far more astounding than these often-cited statistics is that we still do not know *why* many patients suffer from LBP! Not only why, but *how* did the patient develop pack pain, *where* is its origin, *what* caused the problem, and *who* is at risk?

History provides a somber perspective on the diagnosis and treatment of low back pain—and that perspective screams to all clinicians, "be cautious!" In chapter 2 of *Conservative Care of Low Back Pain,*[1] Robert Anderson reviews low back pain diagnoses and treatment since 1800. According to Anderson, in 1850 it was thought that medicine had advanced substantially, although he concludes, "Low back pain fell into a residual category only somewhat less sweepingly inclusive and vague than was the category of arthritis in earlier times." Rheumatism was thought to be the general cause of back pain, originating from irritation in internal organs. Treatments thought to be effective included bleeding, high doses of mercury, narcotics, prolonged bed rest, heat, blistering liniments as a counterirritant, and many others, including galvanism. By 1900, the discovery of infectious microorganisms dominated medical philosophy, thus back pain emerged as an infectious disease. Anderson continues by describing the search for the "focal infection" which would lead to "surgery for tooth extractions, tonsillectomies and adenoidectomies, appendectomies, cholecystectomies, hysterectomies . . . and Lane's operation for removal of the colon." All performed, no doubt, by "skilled clinicians" who *knew* their treatment methods were right. Paul C. Williams, in his classic article entitled "Lesions of the Lumbosacral Spine,"[2] writes: "It is true that infection and congestion play a part and in many cases undoubtedly bring the symptoms into prominence; however, this is true of any mechanically altered articulation which is under strain." Williams wrote that many of the chronic low back patients he saw "gave histories of having had their tonsils and teeth, and occasionally their appendixes, removed."

By 1950, Anderson reports these surgeries were deemed "useless." Spinal surgery instead dominated as the treatment of choice for back pain after research demonstrated that a herniated nucleus pulposus could place pressure on a nerve and cause pain. Anderson reports, "by the 1970s, however, a high incidence of failed surgeries dampened enthusiasm for lumbar spine surgery. It became apparent that probably 99% of back pain patients would not benefit from surgery of any kind." Anderson then encourages the reader by reporting that the 1970s "marked an upturn in the techniques of conservative care. The last quarter of this century witnessed a proliferation of innovative achievements. . . ."

There has been a tremendous increase in the number of conservative therapeutic interventions used today for back pain patients. Innovative treatment techniques in isolation, however, do not bring us closer to solving the problem. Rather, optimism is engendered because low back pain research has proliferated, thus making low back pain treatment a scientific endeavor, though not a successful scientific reality.

The immense quantity of low back pain research over the past 15 years punctuates the seriousness of the search for answers. The Quebec Task Force's report on spinal disorders provides perhaps the most sweeping literary overview to date.[3] Their prominent committee of low back pain scientists identified more than 7,000 articles related to spinal disorders published in the 10 years prior to the report. The number of relevant articles was eventually decreased to 721. The Quebec Task Force reported, "Two hundred fifty-two of the 721 publications were rejected in the evaluation process." A reasonable estimate would be that at least an additional 3,000 articles have been published since 1987. With this vast quantity of research, one would think many answers have been found and, in fact, many have. As highlighted in the monograph from the Quebec Task Force, several treatments for low back pain have been classified as useful, as demonstrated by either randomized or nonrandomized controlled studies. These include short-term bed rest, some systemic medication, electroanalgesia, and exercise. Since that time, further studies have helped mold current philosophies toward back pain management. These include the use of objective feedback during vigorous exercise programs and psychological support, especially for patients with chronic pain.

A great concern is the inappropriate use of both well-controlled and poorly controlled research studies to support clinical opinion. DeRosa and Porterfield, in "A Physical Therapy Model for the Treatment of Low Back Pain"[4] state, "The instructors responsible for orthopedic courses and physical therapy curricula often struggle to introduce the student to a variety of assessment and treatment approaches, even if the various approaches conflict with one another or lack a scientific basis. This diversification of assessment and treatment approaches has occurred simultaneously with the development of new knowledge." The development of varied treatment approaches for back pain has often paralleled new scientific information or new pseudoscientific opinion. Recalling Anderson's comments about low back pain care from the 1850s forward, many thoughts about appropriate treatment were based on small bits of scientific evidence that were subsequently applied, in general terms, to the lumbar spine. Most of these treatments, however, have not withstood scientific scrutiny and have been discarded. Regarding low back pain treatment in the mid-nineteenth century, Anderson states:

> To what extent, then, did a mid-nineteenth century patient profit from conservative measures in the hands of a physician? From a psychological perspective, perhaps it was comforting to place one's health problem in the hands of a doctor. Palliation from rest, heat and mild counter-irritation was offered. . . . Patients suffering from low back pain who avoided physicians probably did better than did those who sought professional care, because only a small part of a doctor's treatment was conservative enough to fit the dictum, "first, do no harm."[1]

Much harm, even today, comes as the result of intervention, not only in the obvious cases of technically poor surgeries performed on the wrong candidates, but also through the confusion and fear instilled in patients, which insidiously leads them to become chronic pain victims. Many diagnostic terms such as *degenerative disc disease* and *degenerative joint disease* promote hopelessness while masking uncertainty. Our egos prevent us from admitting that many times we simply do not understand why a patient continues to suffer from back pain in the presence of "state of the art medical care." The "state of the art" is such that we are often viewed as giving nothing more than palliative care which fosters dependence. Recently, a well-meaning and supportive orthopedic surgeon told me that many times the patients he refers do not have serious pathology but need to "have their hand held."

Are we just holding a patient's hand, or are we applying scientific principles? Are we utilizing diagnostic equipment appropriately, or as a shield to prevent the patient from seeing that we really do not understand? New diagnostic methods are not always that diagnostic. Past age 50, CAT scans are only 50% accurate and, even then, physical signs account for a small portion of the prognostic indicators for successful treatment outcomes.[5,6] As more research is published, we recognize that psychosocial factors contribute prominently to a patient's success or failure with surgery or with conservative care. Unfortunately, conservative therapies rarely develop as the result of scientific scrutiny. Rather, they develop in desperation because old measures have failed, and clinicians can hold onto new treatment methods for 10 or 15 years before discovering that those methods are also worthless. Progress evolves in small increments through the genius of many who labor hard and long to uncover bits of information that may add another piece to an extraordinarily complex puzzle. Clinicians need to embrace research as the validation for their treatment, realizing that not nearly all of the pieces to the puzzle have emerged.

Courses in low back pain management that purport to offer "the solution" and give testimony to miraculous cures take us back to similar statements made a century ago. At the turn of the nineteenth century, nearly all cases of low back pain were labeled as arthritis. Much as a clock that is broken is right twice a day, this diagnosis was also occasionally correct, but not through scientific means. As noted by the Quebec Task Force in chapter 3 of their monograph, "It is generally impossible to corroborate clinical observations through histologic studies, because on one hand the usual benignity of spinal disorders does not justify that tissue be removed and, on the other, there is often no modification of tissue identifiable through current methods." If low back pain diagnosis is not a practical reality for the vast majority of cases, then perhaps LaRocca's statement in the editorial to this monograph captures the real struggle: "The problem emanates from the lack of a comprehensive and unifying problem-solving strategy to appraise the relevant data and from them to establish policy and procedures for implementing effective management while remaining receptive to new learning."[7] Accepting that a solid diagnosis is often impossible, with many diagnoses being verified retrospectively, then the term *diagnosis* should most often be replaced by the term *hypotheses*, and treatment should proceed using clinical algorithms with the end result being successful management of low back pain.

In attending myriad courses, it is impressive to witness support for various diagnostic classification and treatment regimens that in theory are totally in conflict. It seems the more ardent the course instructors' claims of success using specific treatments, the less likely the attendees are to receive an unbiased, scientific accounting of treatment. Nevertheless, it appears that many treatment methods are effective, even when utilizing opposing strategies. What creates their success? Is it simply that most patients are going to get better because low back pain is a relatively benign self-limiting dysfunction, or are we all hitting on some aspect of rehabilitation that is effective? In the movie *Awakenings*, Robin Williams portrays neurologist Dr. Malcolm Sayer treating patients in an undiagnosed, postencephalitic catatonic state. By accident, a patient is given a dose of L-dopa and begins to show signs of improvement. Massive does of L-dopa are then administered and, miraculously, the patients come out of their catatonic states and become functional. Sadly, one by one, each patient gradually slips back into a catatonic state and the elation of the medical staff and family turns to bitter disappointment. Robin Williams then delivers a compassionate soliloquy that applies to all such frustrating endeavors:

> The summer was extraordinary. It was a season of rebirth, an innocence, a miracle; fifteen patients and for us the caretakers. But now we have to adjust to the realities of miracles. We can hide behind the veil of science and say it was the drug that failed, or that the illness itself had returned or that the patients were unable to cope with losing decades of their lives. But the reality is we don't know what went wrong any more than we know what went right. What we do know is as the chemical window closed, another awakening took place. . . . That the human spirit is more powerful than any drug and that is what needs to be nourished. With work, play, friendship, family. These are things that matter—this is what we had forgotten. The simplest things.

We often do not know what goes wrong, and many times we really do not know what goes right. We need to continue validating our clinical practice with scientific information and not become so estranged from research that we risk being fringe practitioners. We have science, we have research, and together with compassion, this is all we have to offer. In the end, win or lose, it is the patients' spirits that need to be nourished. They need to know we care, even if we are unable to help. They need to know that we have given it our best, but that often our best is not good enough. They need to be confident that we know the literature, the research, and the opinions and that we are using these together to their betterment. Let us cling to the dictum "Do no harm." We are moving forward, we are progressing, and we are maturing. As Jules Rothstein states in his editorial to the January 1991 issue of *Physical Therapy:* "As we pass through stages of maturation, our styles and behaviors must change, as must the consequences of our ill-chosen behaviors."[8]

This text is that attempt at a mature approach to back pain rehabilitation. I contend that an accurate diagnosis cannot be the only means of establishing an intelligent management system for patients with low back pain. Many successful models exist without this accurate diagnosis. What is needed is a well-thought-out, research-based orientation to low back pain that allows for our differences in approach but seeks out similarities in treatment method.

References

1. Saal JA, Saal JS: Rehabilitation of the patient, in White AH and Anderson R (eds): Conservative Care of Low Back Pain. Baltimore, Williams and Wilkins, 21–29, 1991.

2. Williams PC: Lesions of the lumbosacral spine, Part I. JBJS 19:343–363, 1937.
3. Spitzer WO, LeBlanc FE, Dupuis M: Scientific approach to the assessment and management of activity-related spinal disorders. Spine 12:7, 1–59, 1987.
4. DeRosa CP, Porterfield JA: A physical therapy model for the treatment of low back pain. Phys Ther 72:4, 261–269, 1992.
5. Wiesel SW, Tsourmas N, Feffer HL, et al: A study of computer-assisted tomography. 1. The incidence of positive CAT scans in an asymptomatic group of patients. Spine 9:549–551, 1984.
6. Lancourt J, Kettehut M: Predicting return to work for lower back pain patients receiving worker's compensation. Spine 17:6, 629–640, 1992.
7. LaRocca H, Editorial in Spitzer WO, LeBlanc FE, Dupuis M: Scientific approach to the assessment and management of activity-related spinal disorders. Spine 12:7, 1–59, 1987.
8. Rothstein JM: The price of maturity (Editorial). Phys Ther 71:1, 1–2, 1991.

I □ □ □
□ □ □
□ □ □

Rehabilitation

Rehabilitation of patients with low back pain (LBP) is a singularly defined process with infinite variety in implementation. Despite varied approaches, clinicians are motivated by a common goal: the restoration of maximum function with minimal symptoms. Over the past three decades, many rehabilitation techniques have emerged in response to this common goal. Without the guidance of controlled clinical trials, however, the efficacy of rehabilitation strategies has been reduced largely to clinical dogma.

The first section of this book examines current clinical philosophies and research related to LBP rehabilitation. Chapter 1, In Search of the Perfect Treatment, examines the major clinical philosophies, highlighting stated differences by drawing from their many commonalities. This chapter systematically explains the many idiosyncratic techniques and customized terminologies which often alienate or intimidate many clinicians. In taking courses from many recognized experts, it becomes clear that philosophies are very divergent, yet the recognized experts' belief in the final outcome is unwavering. Through a systematic process, the mystique of these techniques and terminologies is removed, thereby facilitating an understanding of LBP rehabilitation as an integrated process of not just isolated skills but mature approaches.

The study of different rehabilitation approaches is complicated by individual philosophies regarding the cause of LBP. The complex nature of LBP makes a definitive diagnosis elusive in many cases. Processes need to be developed to guide clinicians through treatment prescriptions. Chapter 2, Exercise Prescription for Low Back Pain, examines specific exercise prescriptions as they relate to LBP. While taking a sports medicine approach and applying it to patients with LBP, the main emphasis is on the decision-making process for exercise prescription. Without specific diagnostic information, exercise prescription must be guided principally by well-defined, clinically observable dysfunctions. In the case of the surgically altered spine, rehabilitation techniques must take into consideration healing times and the nature of the surgical procedure. Rehabilitation for these individuals has largely been empirical as there are no controlled clinical trials to guide the clinician. Chapter 3, Rehabilitation after Back Surgery, explores postsurgical lumbar rehabilitation from the perspective of a noted researcher and orthopedic surgeon.

By viewing LBP rehabilitation as an integrated process of hypothesis-oriented algorithms, the richness of individual approaches will become much clearer and more exciting. In reading this section, the clinician will find the process of rehabilitation to be more easily prescribed while allowing for variations in specific approaches.

1

□ □ □
□ □ □
□ □ □

In Search of the Perfect Treatment

Don Darling

The conservative treatment of lower back pain (LBP) is presently going through rapid changes. In the past, LBP sufferers were advised to take medication, rest in bed for two weeks, "live with the pain," or change occupations. Now they are being treated with mobilization, extension exercises, stabilization programs, back classes, work hardening, myofascial release, strain/counterstrain techniques, and many other active forms of treatment.

Physical therapists are at the forefront of this change in the management of patients who suffer with LBP. Along with this change are some disturbing observations. Physical therapists are attending courses presented by practitioners who appear to be introducing original, new philosophies. These "new" approaches are presented in a manner that portrays the treatment approach as the definitive LBP treatment. Examples of the evaluation and treatment are performed on subjects in front of the class and objective positive results are observed.

Physical therapists return to the clinic feeling they have "found the answer" and that their previous traditional approach was worthless. They use this new philosophy of treatment on their patients only to find that the techniques do not seem to be as effective as they were on the classroom subjects. These therapists then either sign up for the advanced level of the same course to find out more about this treatment approach, or become discouraged and look into other philosophies in their search for a "perfect treatment" approach.

Practitioners may become even more confused when they realize some approaches are completely contradictory. For example, McKenzie extension exercises are used by physical therapists to treat patients with acute LBP. McKenzie has observed that patients with acute LBP lose their lumbar lordosis.[1] His treatment approach attempts to restore their lordosis through exercise and postural principles to relieve their LBP. Conversely, Williams' flexion exercises are also given to patients who have acute LBP. These exercises were designed to reduce the lumbar lordosis which he believed was causing increased compression on the lumbar spine.[2] His treatment approach involved procedures and exercises to reduce the lordotic curve of the lumbar spine. The philosophies of McKenzie and Williams are widely used in the treatment of LBP, yet they appear to be diametrically opposed. This type of discrepancy may be confusing and clinicians will do what they think works best for patients. As a result, therapists have abandoned the use of traditional physical therapy treatment, physical agents, Williams' flexion exercises, and massage for specific treatment philosophies such as craniosacral therapy, strain/counterstrain, or joint-oriented manual therapy.

This chapter will review some common approaches that physical therapists are utilizing in treating the LBP patient. These approaches will be compared critically and a discussion will follow on how they can be integrated into one treatment approach. Further, the chapter will review approaches that have a joint, muscle, or neuromuscular orientation, and a soft tissue approach. Also, psychological aspects and physical agents will be examined as important components of a "perfect treatment" approach for LBP.

Joints

Physical therapists have become more involved in treating LBP patients with joint mobilization. Although the use of mobilization is recent in the field of physical therapy, manual therapy for joints has been used for a long time. Two clinicians who have been instrumental in allowing physical therapists to become involved in joint mobilization and manipulation are John Mennell and James Cyriax.

Mennell

John Mennell is a physician who has written and taught manual medicine techniques for years.[3] He has supported the role of physical therapists in providing joint manipulation to patients who have LBP. Mennell states that all back pathology results in segmental limitation of movement. Back pain cannot be differentiated by the conscious mind to determine whether it is coming from bone, joint, or adjacent levels. The reflex reaction to pain in the back is the splinting of the involved segment of the spine by muscle spasm. Mennell has labeled this condition of the spine *joint dysfunction*. He describes two types of motion that can occur at the joint—voluntary movements and joint play movements.

Normal voluntary movements of the spine are those movements which can occur with normal muscle contraction. Flexion, extension, rotation, and side bending are those voluntary movements that occur at the lumbar spine. Joint play movements are well-defined, very small movements of the joint that allow for easy, painless performance of movement in the voluntary range.[4] Lumbar segmental joint play movements are side tilting, long axis extension, backward tilt, and rotation at the zygapophyseal joints. The loss of spinal joint play movements will be associated with dysfunction and decreased voluntary movements.

Dysfunction is the usual cause of pain in the arthritic joint. Mobilization techniques designed to increase joint play movement at the dysfunctional segment will increase voluntary range of motion and reduce segmental pain.[3] Dysfunction may be caused by trauma, disease, postural defect, preexisting disease, or congenital anomalies. Mennell does not believe the disc plays a significant role in LBP.

Cyriax

James Cyriax was an orthopedist in London who studied and developed a system of evaluation and diagnosis for previously undiagnosed orthopedic problems.[5] Cyriax, contrary to Dr. Mennell, believed that 90% of all lumbar symptoms are attributable to the intervertebral disc. He cites Nachemson's study on disc pressures and postures and concludes that flexion activities and the "flat back" posture increase intradiscal pressure while increasing the lordosis and lying down decrease intradiscal pressure.[6]

Cyriax believed that lumbar muscle strength was of doubtful importance to the prevention of disc injury. He proposed that strengthening muscles may increase the compressive forces on the spine, thus increasing the chance of disc injury. He felt that most back and leg pain was caused by a posterolateral protrusion of the disc placing pressure on the dura mater. This posterior migration of the annular cartilage or nuclear material caused a kyphotic posture. The associated pain and dysfunction caused muscles to contract in order to stabilize the spine and prevent further pain.

Cyriax describes *annular lumbago* as being of quick onset caused by a piece of annular cartilage migrating posteriorly with a flexion activity. *Nuclear lumbago* is a slow onset of LBP after prolonged flexion activities. He treated the annular lumbago with rotation manipulation to put the annular cartilage "back into place." Nuclear lumbago was treated with traction and bed rest. Cyriax advocated immobilization in the lordotic position following successful reduction of the disc.

Cyriax believed that physical agents for the lumbar spine were useless and the only exercises he suggested were passive extension exercises for patients who insisted on doing exercises. Prophylaxis emphasized the importance of maintaining a lordotic posture with activities of daily living. He suggested the use of local epidural anesthesia for lesions that did not respond to manipulation or traction. Cyriax mentioned the rare causes of LBP due to ligamentous stretch, spondylolisthesis, or sacroiliac joint inflammation, but adhered to the belief that the facet joint was not a source of LBP.

Osteopathy

Osteopathy uses a system of healing with an emphasis on manual therapy to treat structural and mechanical problems of the body. The philosophy of osteopathy was first proposed by Andrew Still, a medical doctor in the United States in 1874. The field of osteopathy has undergone significant changes, and, at present, most schools of osteopathy are more similar to medical schools and place little emphasis on manual therapy. Although the traditional osteopaths who still do manual therapy have been known for focusing on the apophyseal joint as the main cause of back pain, osteopathy represents a treatment approach to back pain that applies to the nerves, blood vessels, venous supply, bones, joints, muscles, skin, and connective tissue. Stoddard defines the osteopathic spinal lesion as a condition of impaired mobility in an intervertebral joint.[7] Greenman calls this condition *somatic dysfunction* and defines it as altered function of related components in the somatic (body framework) system: skeletal, arthrodial, and myofascial structures and related vascular, lymphatic, and dural elements. The emphasis of this definition is on altered function of the musculoskeletal system, not on a disease state or pain syndrome.[8]

Greenman uses the mnemonic ART for identifying the area of somatic dysfunction when evaluating the spine. *A* stands for asymmetry of the musculoskeletal system, either structural or functional. *R* represents range of motion alterations of a joint or several joints in the spine. Alteration may be a decrease or an increase in range of motion, although a decrease is the most common observation. *T* is for tissue texture alteration in the soft tissue (skin, fascia, muscle, and ligament).

In evaluating spinal joint dysfunction, Greenman looks at apophyseal joint mechanics and positional changes to assess restrictions in the opening and closing of the apophyseal joints. He describes two types of spinal dysfunction. Type I involves three or more segments of the lumbar spine with minimal forward or backward bending restriction. Most of the restriction is in side bending and rotation to the opposite side of the side bending restriction. In other words, on palpation of the transverse processes one may assess decreased mobility in left rotation (a fullness on the right side) and right side bending (concavity on the left side) that does not change appreciably with flexion or extension.

A Type II (non-neutral) restriction involves a single motion segment and includes significant restriction into flexion or extension. The motion restriction involves limitation of side bending and rotation to the same side. In other words, if the patient has a Type II restriction at L4–5 in which the facet joint is unable to close (backward bending of the spine), the patient would exhibit a fullness on the left side when in extension and this would indicate the segment is unable to extend, right side bend, and right rotate. When the patient flexes, the asymmetry should be less because both facet joints have opened. Based on this type of evaluation, joint manipulation can be carried out to promote closing of the right facet joint, increasing extension, and resolving the joint component of that somatic dysfunction.

A Type I (neutral) dysfunction usually occurs in conjunction with a Type II dysfunction. For example, if a patient has a limitation at L4–5 into backward bending, right side bending, and right rotation, a Type I group dysfunction may be cephalad to L4–5 with significant limitation of left side bending and right rotation. Although this is a simple system of mechanics and subsequent treatment, there are no studies that substantiate the validity and reliability of this approach. Assessment of spinal mobility based on static positional diagnosis may give incorrect information if the patient has bony anomalies, altered facet joint angles, or if there is a difference in muscle tone or muscle mass.

The assessment of somatic dysfunction may accompany many other diagnoses or may be present as an independent entity. The osteopathic approach emphasizes evaluating the dysfunction, correlating it with clinical symptoms, and treating the dysfunction to promote normal mobility, strength, and coordination, resulting in prolonged relief of LBP. It is interesting to note that many manual therapy approaches being taught today by physical therapists have their roots in osteopathy.

Maitland

Geoffrey Maitland, a physiotherapist from Australia, has developed a system of mobilization and manual therapy which focuses on the patient's subjective complaints and the quality of pain. This approach to LBP is now used by many physical therapists throughout the world.[9] Maitland places great emphasis on the patient's pain, behavior of the pain, and subjective response to different types of passive movements or changes in position. He advises the avoidance of "diagnostic titles" to prevent confusion. He does not use manipulation exclusively.

According to Maitland there are three important aspects of manual therapy that can make it an effective tool in the treatment of LBP. First, the treating therapist must do continuous analytical assessments throughout the treatment. Second, the initial application of a technique must be gentle. Third, the symptomatic responses both before and after the patient's treatment must be assessed and analyzed before progressing. He states that "manipulation is not like a game of golf where the player uses a technique to hit a ball in the direction he wants it to go . . . manipulation is more like a game of chess where different pieces can be moved in many different and specific ways, and where plans are made and destroyed and changed until the goal is achieved."[9] The way these pieces are moved may be changed by how the opponent (patient) responds to these moves, thus each chess game (treatment) is completely different depending on the moves of the opponent.

Using this analogy, Maitland describes the importance of assessing pain in response to initial examination and treatment techniques and adjusting the treatment program throughout the assessment. When symptoms are easily produced, techniques may be chosen to either relieve or provoke these symptoms.

Maitland divides joint mobility into two different types—physiological and accessory. Physiological movements are those movements the patient can perform actively. Physiological movements of the lumbar spine are flexion, extension, lateral flexion, and rotation. Accessory movements of a joint cannot be produced actively, but can be produced by another person. These are similar to the joint play movements that Mennell has described. Accessory movements in the lumbar spine are created by posteroanterior central vertebral pressure, posteroanterior unilateral vertebral pressure, transverse vertebral pressure, and longitudinal traction. Maitland emphasizes the importance of communication and documentation of techniques used in treatment. He has developed a system of four grades of passive movements. Grade I is a small amplitude movement near the starting position of the range. Grade II is a large amplitude movement which carries well into the range that is free of any stiffness or spasm. Grade III is also a large amplitude movement, but goes into the stiffness and muscle spasm (end range). Grade IV is a small amplitude movement stretching into the stiffness or muscle spasm.

Maitland has also developed a system of recording manual techniques. Posteroanterior unilateral vertebral pressure on the left would be recorded as $\sqrt{}^{\bullet}$ or transverse vertebral pressure to the right would be recorded as →. A system to record movement at a particular joint has also been developed by Maitland. This system records range of motion, pain, resistance, and muscle spasm. Although it is complicated, this system can be used as a valuable tool in recording a patient's progress and communicating results with other physical therapists.

In summary, Maitland has developed a system of evaluation and treatment that focuses on a patient's subjective description of pain and subjective response to manual treatment. Since he relies on subjective description, a system of recording treatment techniques and the patient's responses to the techniques applied has been developed. Less emphasis is placed on normal arthrokinematics, ability to perform functional activities, and self-treatment through individualized exercise programs and general fitness.

McKenzie

Robin McKenzie is a physical therapist from New Zealand who has developed an approach to LBP which emphasizes self-treatment. He states that 70% to 75% of all patients who suffer from LBP should be able to treat themselves and do not need mobilization or specific hands-on treatment.[1] McKenzie believes that all patients should see a medical doctor for a medical diagnosis before being evaluated by a physical therapist for mechanical treatment. He calls his approach the "prophylactic technique" and describes three predisposing factors that cause low back pain: sitting posture, limited range of motion into extension, and the predominance of flexion activities in our society. Simply stated, lumbar flexion is the predisposing factor for most back problems. He divides back problems into three distinct syndromes: postural, dysfunction, and derangement.

The postural syndrome occurs when abnormal forces are placed on normal structures. For example, prolonged seated flexion places abnormal stress on the intervertebral disc and posterior elements. With prolonged stretching of these structures the patient may notice back pain. When the patient's posture changes from a flexed position to a lordotic position, the pain is immediately relieved.

In the dysfunction syndrome, pain may be caused by either normal or abnormal stresses being placed on abnormal tissue. This may be soft tissue that has sustained a previous injury and is scarred into a shortened position, or soft tissue that has adaptively shortened in response to a prolonged, altered posture. The treatment of dysfunction is administered by exercising and stretching the restriction in a graded manner that does not increase the pain. Therefore, if a patient is unable to perform lumbar flexion, graded flexion exercises are prescribed that decrease LBP with repetition and increase pain-free flexibility.

In the derangement syndrome, McKenzie theorizes that back and leg pain are caused from the posterior migration of the nucleus pulposis. This change in position can decrease the mobility of the intervertebral motion segment and limit the ability of the spine to backward bend. The fluid usually shifts in a posterolateral direction causing the patient to assume a flexed and laterally shifted posture away from the painful side. The pain is caused by mechanical irritation to the nociceptors in the posterior longitudinal ligament, outer fibers of the annulus fibrosis, or the ventral aspect of the dura mater.[1] A derangement may be progressive, starting as back pain and "peripheralizing" into the leg as it gets worse. McKenzie describes the "centralization phenomena" in which movements of the spine (usually passive extension) will cause less leg pain and at times increase the pain in the mid-lumbar area. McKenzie suggests that this phenomena is explained by the nucleus pulposis being pushed anteriorly, thus reducing the disc bulge. Although there are no studies that support the theory of a shift in the nucleus pulposis with a change in posture, studies have been performed on the clinical effectiveness of the McKenzie approach.

Donelson and his colleagues evaluated eighty-seven LBP patients who also had pain radiating into the buttock, thigh, or calf.[10] These patients were evaluated and treated by a physical therapist trained in the "McKenzie techniques." Donelson found that rapid centralization of symptoms occurred in 87% of these patients; 83% of the overall patient group recorded good to excellent results from treatment. Of the patients with excellent results, 100% had exhibited centralization of symptoms at the initial evaluation. Donelson also found in the group of patients who had back pain for 0 to 4 weeks that 98% achieved good to excellent results. Six patients in this group did not centralize their pain and three actually had peripheralization of the pain. Four of the six patients went on to surgery with excellent results 3 to 5 years postoperatively.

McKenzie, like Cyriax, believes that 95% of lower back pain comes from the intervertebral disc. There are no experimental studies that confirm this theory.

Contrary to what many practitioners think, McKenzie exercises are not limited to lumbar extension. His approach utilizes a detailed, simple evaluation that involves active and passive movements and records the patient's subjective pain response to the movements. Based on evaluation results, the patient is given a home exercise program to decrease pain. Therefore, if flexion is found to decrease or centralize pain, the patient is given flexion exercises, reevaluated and treated accordingly. Reevaluation may reveal that the patient's syndrome has changed. Derangement syndrome, for example, may progress into a dysfunction syndrome and exercises will be changed accordingly. Pain with flexion and deviation to the side of the pain that improves with repetition could represent a dysfunction syndrome and indicate that the patient needs to stretch into this position. The patient can be instructed in graded exercises that will allow stretching into the position of limitation without increasing pain.

When the patient does not respond to self-treatment techniques, hands-on mobilization may be indicated. McKenzie demonstrates five mobilization techniques for these patients which he states comprise 25% to 30% of all patients with LBP. These techniques involve extension mobilization, rotation and flexion, and rotation and extension. These techniques can be combined with self-exercise and individualized body mechanics instruction to provide effective long-term management of patients with LBP.

Paris

Stanley Paris is a physiotherapist from New Zealand who has developed a philosophy of treatment based on the work of Cyriax, Mennell, and Stoddard.[11] He has been instrumental in developing and promoting the field of orthopedic physical therapy in the United States. He notes that 80% of patients with LBP get better no matter what type of treatment is rendered. He suggests treatment be concentrated toward the 20% of patients who do not get better within two weeks.

Paris describes two types of movement that occur at joints—classical and accessory. Classical movements are defined as osteokinematic movements which involve the change in the angle of the limbs. Examples of classical movements are shoulder abduction or lumbar flexion. Classical movements may be performed actively by the individual's own efforts or passively by an outside force such as manual stretching.

Paris describes two types of accessory movements. Component motions of a joint are the arthrokinematic movements that take place within a joint. These are the roll, slide, and spin that add up to an active motion. Joint play is another accessory motion that takes place in the joint in response to an outside force. Paris defines joint manipulation as a skilled passive movement directed at joint accessory motions.[11] Joint manipulation is divided into three subtypes: distraction provides separation of the bony elements; nonthrust utilizes stretch, oscillations, and isometric contraction; and thrust employs high-speed, short-amplitude motion of the joint.

The Paris philosophy focuses on the evaluation and appropriate treatment of joint function.[12] He describes a joint injury as a dysfunction and not a disease. With decreased mobility, the treatment indicated is manipulation to the joint, stretching of the muscles and fascia, and promotion of activities to increase full flexibility. If hypermobility is present, manipulation to adjacent hypomobile segments, along with stabilization exercises and teaching correct body mechanics, is indicated. Once normal function returns, the underlying mechanical cause of the patient's pain will be eliminated, thereby decreasing the chance of a recurring episode.

Paris performs a detailed mechanical evaluation of the spine focusing on intersegmental function. The mechanical evaluation is thought to assess zygapophyseal joint mechanics as does the osteopathic approach. Paris has found that virtually all spinal structures can be involved in dysfunction and disease and are capable of causing pain. Paris advocates looking at syndromes versus trying to determine a specific diagnosis regarding which structure is causing the pain. By working with these syndromes, Paris states, he has become successful in selecting the best treatment approach for each syndrome. His approach requires practice, time, and education to obtain the skills necessary to treat each individual syndrome.

Paris contends that most acute pain in the lower back is from an injury to the zygapophyseal joint capsule. The resulting pain can cause stiffness, muscle guarding, and decreased nutrition to the joint. Joint manipulation is the treatment of choice to promote normal arthrokinematics and prevent further injury to the back.

In summary, physical therapists have become more involved in the manual treatment of joint dysfunction of the lumbar spine. It appears the roots of manual therapy are in both the osteopathic approach and in the teachings of James Cyriax and John Mennell. Physical therapists have taken these concepts even further. The approaches of McKenzie and Maitland focus more on the patient's subjective complaints in response to manual treatment. McKenzie has taken Cyriax's work and developed it to more of a self-management technique which involves exercise, self-treatment, and education. The osteopathic approach and Stanley Paris's approach place more emphasis on evaluating the normal mechanics of the spine, observing that the patient's pain complaints will diminish as function improves. All of these approaches emphasize a specific evaluation which determines treatment choices.

Although joint mobilization and self-mobilization can be effective in the management of patients with LBP, there are many other structures that contain nociceptors and can cause significant LBP. The next section will review approaches that emphasize the soft tissue component of LBP.

Soft Tissue

Trigger Points

A common diagnosis associated with LBP is *muscle strain.* Many patients report they feel as though they have a "pulled muscle." Janet Travell, M.D., and David Simons, M.D., have developed a general approach to the diagnosis and treatment of LBP, emphasizing the muscle as the primary cause of LBP.[13] They define painful muscles as having myofascial trigger points which are self-sustaining, hyperirritable foci causing local and referred pain. A mechanical strain to the muscle may initiate the trigger point activity and mechanical or systemic factors such as a short leg or vitamin D deficiency can perpetuate the problem.

Travell believes the myofascial component of LBP should be first treated with passive stretching combined with a vapocoolant sprayed over the involved muscle. If this does not help, an injection into the trigger point is recommended. Travell also advocates ischemic compression to the trigger point along with stretching and strengthening exercises. She acknowledges that joint dysfunction may be a perpetuating factor in LBP, but places emphasis on treatment of the myofascial pain component.

Muscle Imbalances

Shirley Sahrmann has added to the principles of Florence Kendall in evaluating the muscles' role in LBP.[14,15] She looks for postural imbalance along with specific muscle imbalances which may increase stresses on the musculoskeletal system and cause pain. Kendall and Sahrmann's philosophy is to change faulty alignment by achieving musculoskeletal balance. Sahrmann defines two types of muscle imbalances—passive muscle imbalance, in which a muscle is too weak or not active, and active muscle imbalance, in which one muscle in a group of synergistic muscles predominates and overpowers the other muscles. For example, during hip abduction in the side lying position, increased hip flexion with external rotation may result from increased tensor fascia lata activity which overpowers the gluteus medius and gluteus minimus. Sahrmann believes that the proper sequence in correcting muscle imbalances is to first increase the strength of the weakened muscle. She advocates the use of "muscle training" to make sure the patient is contracting the right muscles in the correct sequence when performing the home exercise program.

Vladimir Janda is a Czechoslovakian physiatrist who has studied the response of muscles to chronic pain and dysfunction. He has discovered that certain muscles become tight in response to pain and has labeled these "tonic muscles" (Table 1.1). Other muscles consistently become weak in response to pain; these are called "phasic muscles" (Table 1.2). Janda believes, as do other researchers, that primary and traumatic muscle lesions have a doubtful place in the etiology of acute lumbar pain, but muscle imbalances may develop in response to an injury to the disc, ligaments, or zygapophyseal joints. The acute pain from the injury causes the muscle to respond in the observed manner. If the pain is not treated effectively, the muscle imbalances remain. Muscles that are tight become activated easily and may cause weakness to their antagonist due to reciprocal inhibition.

Table 1.1   Muscles with Mainly Postural (Tonic) Function

Quadratus lumborum

Back extensors
  Erector Spinae
  Longissimus thoracis
  Rotators
  Multifidus

Hip flexors
  Iliopsoas
  Tensor fascia latae
  Rectus femoris

Lateral rotators of the hip
  Piriformis

Medial rotators of the hip
  Pectineus
  Adductor longus
  Adductor brevis
  Adductor magnus

Hamstrings
  Biceps femoris
  Semitendinosus
  Semimembranosus

Plantar flexors
  Gastrocnemius
  Soleus
  Tibialis posterior

Table 1.2   Muscles with Mainly Dynamic (Phasic) Function

Rectus abdominus

Obliquus externus abdominis

Obliquus internus abdominis

Gluteus minimus, gluteus medius, gluteus maximus

Vastus medialis and lateralis

Tibialis anterior

Peronei

These muscle imbalances may then become a perpetuating factor of postural imbalance, joint dysfunction, and chronic mechanical pain.

Janda has observed that after stretching a tight muscle the antagonist spontaneously becomes much stronger. Thus he believes, contrary to Sahrmann, that tight muscles should be stretched before starting a strengthening program. Janda and Sahrmann do agree that a detailed evaluation is required to allow for specific instruction and training in the appropriate exercise program.

Lewitt agrees with Janda's view of muscle imbalances and pain. He believes that tension on ligaments, fascia, and joint capsules is the source of much LBP.[17] The tension may be caused by physical imbalances or psychological input. The most frequent cause of tension is disturbed neuromuscular function. Lewitt emphasizes the role of the nervous system in treating painful low back syndromes. Therefore, therapists should not only be evaluating the involved muscle for pain, tightness, or weakness, but should also evaluate the correct sequence of contraction of these muscles and look for smooth eccentric contraction. The pain may not be coming from primary muscle pathology but may be due to mechanical pain in joints, ligaments, or capsules because the muscles are not coordinating to support these structures and allow for normal arthrokinematic movement.

Neuromuscular System

Physical therapy has historically been associated with rehabilitation and the use of rehabilitation techniques for the neurologically involved patient. Many techniques originally developed for the neurologically impaired patient are now being used for patients with LBP. Proprioceptive neuromuscular facilitation (PNF) is an approach to rehabilitation based on the work of Sherrington who first defined the concept of muscle facilitation and inhibition.[18] Herman Kabat, M.D., Ph.D., a physician and neurophysiologist, developed rehabilitation techniques based on Sherrington's work. Margaret Knott, a physical therapist, worked with Dr. Kabat and developed the principles of PNF in the rehabilitation of her neurological patients.[19] She developed many specific techniques, but emphasized the principles over the techniques. The program involves functional patterns that the patient learns. The therapist uses different types of proprioceptive input to facilitate the desired muscular activity and inhibit undesirable activity. These techniques use manual pressure, compression, or traction of the joints. Ideally, the program progresses to allow the patient to perform the exercises independently.

Berta Bobath, an English physical therapist, has developed a system of neuromuscular reeducation in the treatment of patients who have had strokes. Some of her principles and techniques have been adapted to the treatment of LBP. Bobath examines normal reciprocal interaction of muscles with rehabilitation and notes alteration in normal eccentric contraction with elongation against gravity, as well as observing cocontraction of muscles. This phenomena can be observed in patients with LBP who are unable to forward bend smoothly or extend their lumbar spine from the fully flexed position without using their hands to help due to the altered reciprocal inhibition between agonist and antagonist.[17,20]

Muscle Energy Technique

Muscle energy technique is a system developed by Mitchell, an osteopathic physician. He combines the neurophysiological principles of Sherrington with the osteopathic principles of joint biomechanics and arthrokinematics.[21] The techniques, as applied to the spine, involve positioning a segment at the end of its restriction and having the patient actively contract the shortened muscle isometrically. After contraction, the tight muscle can be stretched. Muscle energy technique can also be utilized with the patient contracting the antagonist of the shortened muscle thus causing relaxation of the tight muscle and strengthening the weakened muscle through reciprocal inhibition. The movements are done in three planes or in a diagonal. This approach is very similar to PNF. Philip Greenman, D.O., believes muscle energy technique is the most valuable form of manual therapy, effecting changes in joint, muscle length, muscle strength, and tightened fascia while removing passive congestion and promoting normal function.[8]

Functional Technique

Functional technique is another osteopathic approach to treatment based on restoring normal muscle coordination and joint mobility to a segment.[8] These procedures focus on evaluating the quality of motion more than quantity. The treatment theory is that abnormal afferent activity is coming from an area of dysfunction due to stimulation of nociceptors. Functional techniques try to restore proper afferent signals through the positioning and monitoring of a segment where there is least resistance and greatest comfort. This would be classified as an indirect technique in which the joint is mobilized in the opposite direction of the restriction. Direct techniques are those in which the barrier is engaged and stretched. In using functional techniques the therapist helps the patient find the most comfortable position and monitors changes by palpating the area of tenderness. This is similar to the "strain/counterstrain" techniques used by Jones to position and hold the joint in its most comfortable position while palpating muscle tone.[22] He concurrently assesses the change in mobility and function and neuromuscular coordination.

Massage

Massage is one of the first manual tools taught in physical therapy school. There are as many different approaches to massage as there are people who practice massage. Mary McMillan is one of the key people who promulgated massage among physical therapists as the field grew in the early 1900s.[23] Although massage has been used for thousands of years, it continues to grow as a popular form of treatment. Some systems use massage over acupuncture points or trigger points such as in accupressure or shiatsu. Bonnie Pruden has developed a system utilizing deep massage over trigger points based on input from Hans Kraus, Janet Travell, and Desmond Tivy.[24] Other systems evaluate the role of abnormal posture and movement in LBP, seeking to reorganize and balance the body in response to gravitational forces. Rolf uses a system of pressure points and stretch techniques in a precise sequence to effect physical function and change in posture.[24]

John Mennell has stated there are two effects of massage—mechanical and reflexive.[25] Massage to the dehydrated connective tissue stimulates production of ground substances, assists in the orientation of collagen fibers, and breaks fibrofatty microadhesions. Further mobilization can result in plastic deformation of connective tissue increasing extensibility, length, and mobility. Massage may also cause reflexive effects from stimulation of sensory receptors in the skin and subcutaneous tissue. The stimuli pass along afferent fibers of the peripheral nervous system to the spinal cord. From there stimuli may be dispersed through the central and autonomic nervous systems, producing effects such as capillary vasodilatation or constriction, relaxation or stimulation of voluntary muscle, sedation or stimulation of sensory receptors, and relief.[23,26]

Massage can be a valuable tool, whether focusing on pain or improving function. It can be used in conjunction with muscle stretching and muscle coordination exercises to promote healing or decrease pain.

Myofascial Release

Myofascial release is largely an osteopathic technique used by some physical therapists. Ward describes myofascial release as a bridging technique spanning the spectrum of manual therapy.[8] Myofascial release may be used in a direct or indirect technique. Greenman reports four basic concepts of myofascial release techniques. The first is the "tight/loose" concept. Tightness causes asymmetry and looseness allows asymmetry. The second concept is the importance of palpation. The third is the neuroreflexive change that occurs with manual force on the musculoskeletal system. The fourth is the release phenomena that occurs with manual force. The goal of myofascial release is not only to increase mobility and strength, but to enhance muscle coordination.

Upledger notes that the majority of fascial planes are oriented longitudinally in the body.[27] Gliding mobility is more noticeable in the longitudinal direction. Anatomically, there are specific structures that restrict longitudinal movement. These occur where there is an increase in transverse soft tissue. Upledger identifies four areas where restrictions can occur: the respiratory diaphragm, pelvic diaphragm, thoracic inlet, and the cranial base. Manual treatment involves moving the fascia in three planes to allow for a release. Upledger promotes using very gentle force with the hands above and below the areas identified as restricted. Too much force is counterproductive. The placement of the hands should allow for shearing, torsion, and rotation and the force should not return in the same direction. The therapist should sense softening or release with gentle pressure. When therapists first utilize these techniques, they may not feel they are being effective in their treatment. Myofascial release can be useful in treating a patient who is acute or who is not comfortable with "hands-on" therapy. Myofascial release can allow the patient to get accustomed to manual treatment and thus the treatment can progress to a more direct approach. Myofascial release appears to be effective due to its reflexive effects on the central nervous system, not to the physical changes of the soft tissue.

Craniosacral Technique

Craniosacral technique was developed by William Garner Sutherland, D.O., as an extension of Andrew Still's principles of articulation of the cranium.[28] Sutherland believed he was able to palpate movement between the sutures of the cranium. He hypothesized that the cranium of the healthy individual would have normal mobility between the sutures, but restrictions or altered mobility would be palpated during times of ill health. Sutherland reported palpating a "primary respiratory mechanism" in the craniosacral system which occurs 10 to 14 times per minute with low amplitude.[28] The rhythm reportedly is not associated with heart rate, breathing, or alpha rhythm of the brain. Upledger compares the craniosacral system to a semiclosed hydraulic system. He states that this system is related closely to the central nervous system, autonomic nervous system, the neuromuscular skeletal system, and the endocrine system. The dura mater is the outside boundary of this system and is impermeable to the cerebrospinal fluid it holds. The craniosacral system obeys the laws of fluid dynamics. Pressure over the fluids, whether in the cranial or sacral area transmits force equally in all directions. This characteristic makes the craniosacral system amenable to "shotgun" types of treatment.[8] The craniosacral system proceeds through cyclical flexion and extension at the rate of 6 to 12 cycles per second.[27] During the flexion phase, the whole body externally rotates and the head widens. During the extension phase the whole body internally rotates and the head narrows in an anterior/posterior axis. Restrictions and changes in inherent motion are assessed through very light palpation. Treatment is administered very gently in an indirect manner (away from the barrier) or a direct manner (into the restricted barrier). Greenman states that dysfunction of the craniosacral system may be primary or secondary. Cranial dysfunction may be the result of alteration elsewhere in the musculoskeletal system. Greenman has stated that if the musculoskeletal component is not treated appropriately, results of other manual therapy will be diminished. Conversely, continued attention to the musculoskeletal system elsewhere without addressing craniosacral dysfunction may also allow for less-than-satisfactory results.

In summary, the neuromuscular component in the treatment of LBP is an important aspect in management of these patients. Physical therapists have many approaches they can use in the treatment of patients ranging from traditional physical therapy rehabilitation techniques, PNF and NDT, to passive stretching, coordination exercises, and fluoromethane spray and stretch techniques. Other neuromuscular techniques such as myofascial release and craniosacral technique that have come from the osteopaths may also be an effective component in the overall mechanical treatment of LBP.

Traditional Physical Therapy

There is a current trend away from the use of passive modalities for the treatment of LBP with the focus being placed on active, mechanical, and what is perceived to be more substantive physical therapy treatment.[29,30] Physical modalities have helped patients in the past and can be a valuable adjunct in effective treatment. Modalities may accelerate the rate of healing and help achieve the goal of independence at a faster pace. Modalities may be used to decrease pain, promote healing, increase extensibility of tightened structures, and improve muscle coordination.[30] Ice may be used in the acute phase to limit the extravasation of blood from the damaged vessels to the tissues by constricting blood vessels, and later with reflexive vasodilitation may promote removal of chemicals causing pain in muscles. Cold can also decrease muscle guarding. Heat can increase the circulation to the area, increasing extensibility of the collagen to help control pain. Ultrasound can mechanically heat deep structures and promote healing. There are various forms of electric stimulation that have effects of reducing pain, decreasing swelling, promoting healing, increasing strength, decreasing inflammation, and promoting normal firing patterns of the muscles, as well as decreasing muscle spasm.[30] It is important to note that physical agents should be administered along with a mechanical treatment program that promotes independent management of the low back problem.

The decision to use physical modalities should be based on the evaluation with specific goals in mind. If the soft tissues are more flexible after being heated, the patient's pain level is less, making manual therapy to hypomobile joints and passive stretching to tightened soft tissue more effective. It can also help patients psychologically. If they feel better after treatment, they may be more motivated to follow through with their home exercise program. A TENS unit may enable patients to do their exercises on a more regular basis and also may decrease the effect of pain on altered muscle firing patterns, thus promoting normal function in the area.

Exercise

Another traditional realm of physical therapy is exercise to treat LBP. There is recent evidence that people who are physically fit and exercise regularly have a decreased incidence of LBP.[31,32] For this reason, exercise and fitness instruction should be part of the treatment program for patients with LBP. It is important that this program should start as soon as possible to minimize the effects of immobility. The Norwegians identify three major categories of exercise in promoting physical fitness: cardiorespiratory capacity and efficiency, muscle strength and endurance, and flexibility.[33] They have developed a system that works major muscle groups in sequence to benefit muscular strength, muscular endurance, and flexibility. They have three levels or sequences of exercises that can be done without the use of weights, three levels with conventional weights, and exercises that can be done with specific exercise equipment. Sequence 1 exercises duplicate many of the motions that occur with the activities of daily living.

Tom Mayer has adapted the "sports medicine approach" to the lumbar spine and advocates active management of LBP patients.[29] His first phase of active management starts with stretching and flexibility exercises. The second phase focuses on strength, endurance, and aerobic capacity, assuming that most of the mobility problems have been resolved. As patients improve, the exercise program can be modified to include movements or postures that simulate the specific activities they need to perform their normal daily routines.

In his review of the literature on neural adaptation to resistance training Sale found that early increases in strength are associated mainly with neural adaptation from improved coordination, learning, or increased activation of the primary mover muscles.[34] Therefore, specificity should be a part of all exercise programs for patients with LBP. This type of specific training can provide a safety margin to prevent reinjury to the back when patients return to normal activity. This treatment can also build confidence and morale for patients who are unsure of their ability to return to their work. Patients may require a work hardening program if their functional capacity cannot be elevated to a level where they can return to work. This involves patients doing job tasks under supervision. At this stage in rehabilitation, it is important that the therapist communicate with other professionals regarding the patients' job requirements and specific needs in order for them to return to work. With appropriate communication, all professionals involved can focus on the same realistic goals to return patients to daily activities that will not exacerbate their LBP.

Psychology of Lower Back Pain

One of the greatest handicaps for a practitioner treating LBP is the lack of knowledge regarding the patient's psychosocial history and emotional reaction to LBP. Barry Wyke defines pain as an emotional response to nociceptive input.[35] In other words, pain is not a primary sense such as sight, hearing, or smell. It is more an emotional reaction to nociception. Therefore, how patients respond to pain depends on their personality and emotional state. Emotional state should be a factor in determining the type of treatment a patient will receive.

John Sarno, M.D., has emphasized the emotional component of pain and has described a disorder called tension myositis syndrome.[37] He describes a benign but painful disorder caused by tension in the muscles that is not due to physical or mechanical irritation but is caused by the emotional process. He notes there is wide acceptance that gastric ulcers are caused by emotional tension. Similarly, nerves and tender ligaments can be affected by emotional tension which can decrease blood flow to muscles, nerves, tendons, and ligaments. Decreased blood flow can cause chemical and mechanical nociception in the muscles.

Sarno treats pain patients by informing them that they are having an emotional problem that is causing tension and pain. The patients attend two 2-hour sessions. The first session educates in the physiology and diagnosis of tension myositis syndrome; the second reviews the psychology of tension myositis and the treatment for it. Sarno tells the patients not to worry because it is a harmless problem, they should renew their normal physical activity, discontinue any type of physical treatment for their problem, and focus on the psychological, not the physical. He goes through a long list of LBP diagnoses that he feels are mainly caused by tension myositis syndrome. Dr. Sarno does not have any hard data to prove the effectiveness of his program. It is interesting to read several of his case studies in which patients who have long histories of back pain and dysfunction experience significant relief of the problem after the 2-hour sessions. It appears that when patients understand the causes of their back pain, they become less apprehensive about their problem and are able to go on living with it.

Summary

The first part of this chapter briefly reviewed current approaches to the treatment of LBP. Each can take years of study and practice to perfect. After reviewing these approaches, several common components appear to be important to their success. Most of these philosophies do not view LBP as one overall diagnosis that is treated with the same regime for all patients. They emphasize the importance of an evaluation to determine what specific type of treatment is indicated for the patient. Most of these evaluations involve *listening* to the patient describe the onset and behavior of the pain. The evaluation also includes *observation* of the painful area. Many of these approaches encourage palpation to the area that is painful. By listening carefully to the patient describe the problem and correlating this with an objective evaluation, the treating physical therapist should be able to administer an effective individualized program. Many patients with chronic LBP will report that this is the first time someone has taken the time to assess their pain or even touch the area of pain. It is not surprising that these patients have not had previous successful treatment and now exhibit chronic pain behavior.

Another common factor that binds the different treatment approaches together is that *something* concrete is being done to deal with the patient's LBP. The patient is being touched, moved, and actively participating in a program with specific short-term and long-term goals. This in itself can relieve emotional stress which could be a perpetuating factor of the patient's pain.

There are also many similarities in actual treatment techniques for patients with LBP, although the different approaches purport to target different structures. For example, working on correcting a right lateral shift using the McKenzie technique, reportedly for a herniated disc at L4–5 to the left side (Figure 1.1) is similar to the movement used in the osteopathic approach when treating a Type II non-neutral dysfunction at L4–5. The latter presumes a limitation in backward bending, left side bending, and left rotation due to limited left zygapophyseal joint mobility into extension (Figure 1.2). If the patient were standing in a right lateral shift a muscle spasm may occur in the right quadratus lumborum with a palpable trigger point in this area. Travell would suggest spray and stretch in the left side bent position with the spine in slight extension (Figure 1.3). These three treatment maneuvers require almost identical positioning for the patient. They probably are affecting all three structures in a similar manner.

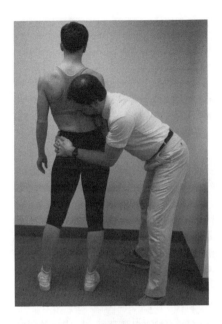

Figure 1.1 Working on correcting a right lateral shift using the McKenzie technique, reportedly for a herniated disc at L4–5 to the left side.

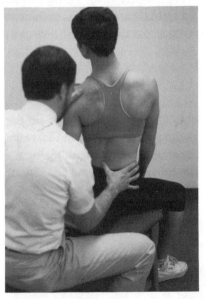

Figure 1.2 Osteopathic approach when treating a Type II non-neutral dysfunction at L4–5. This approach presumes a limitation in backward bending, left side bending, and left rotation due to limited left zygapophyseal joint mobility into extension.

Another similarity between treatment approaches would occur in the patient with a posteriorly rotated left ilium, complaining of pain in the left lower back and hip area. In the joint-oriented approach, the patient would be treated with passive mobilization to promote anterior rotation of the right ilium as shown in Figure 1.4. In the Janda muscle approach, passive stretch of the rectus femoris and psoas would be indicated in the technique as shown in

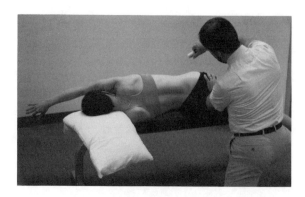

Figure 1.3 Spray and stretch in the left side bent position with the spine in slight extension.

Figure 1.5. When evaluating a patient utilizing Shirley Sahrmann's muscle imbalance approach, the patient may exhibit an altered muscle firing pattern in the gluteus maximus and specific strengthening exercises would be indicated, working on active hip extension. All three of these activities involve the same type of movement but purport to be treating different structures. If a patient is being stretched, using a slump stretch as described by Maitland to stretch tightened dura or an adherent nerve root (Figure 1.6), this would be very similar to Travell stretching the lumbar paraspinal musculature with fluoromethane spray and stretch techniques in the forward bent position (Figure 1.7).

The Perfect Treatment

After studying philosophies of LBP management, their similarities and their differences, it is easy to be confused about how an individual practitioner can develop an objective treatment approach. The following section will attempt to develop a "perfect treatment approach" based on clinical

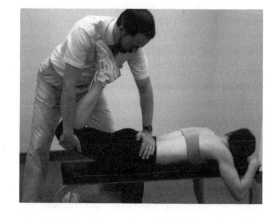

Figure 1.4 Treatment of the patient with a posteriorly rotated left ilium, complaining of pain in the left lower back and hip area. In the joint-oriented approach, the patient would be treated with passive mobilization to promote anterior rotation of the right ilium as shown.

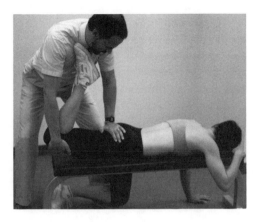

Figure 1.5 Treatment of the patient with a posteriorly rotated left ilium, complaining of pain in the left lower back and hip area. In the Janda muscle approach, passive stretch of the rectus femoris and psoas would be indicated in the technique as shown.

philosophies presented in this chapter. Nonclinical but important components of a treatment approach will also be presented.

The initial LBP evaluation is the single most important component toward developing appropriate, effective treatment for the patient. Most people would agree that the term LBP is not a diagnosis. Prescribing the same program for every person with LBP would be similar to a medical doctor prescribing the same treatment for everyone who presents with abdominal pain. A patient with LBP must be evaluated to find what structures are painful, what positions increase and decrease pain, and what factors may be perpetuating the chronic irritation. Evaluation of the patient with LBP will tell the practitioner if the patient is acute, subacute, or chronic. If the patient is acute, conventional modalities may be indicated to relieve pain and promote healing. Although it is difficult to identify the specific structure or structures causing the patient's pain, the evaluation should give an idea of

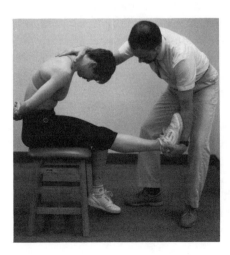

Figure 1.6 Using a slump stretch approach described by Maitland to stretch tightened dura or an adherent nerve root.

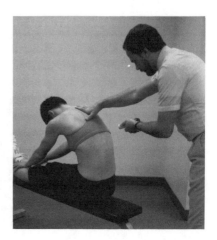

Figure 1.7 Stretching the lumbar paraspinal musculature with fluoromethane spray and stretch techniques in the forward bent position.

what structures may be primarily involved. If the evaluation reveals that the pain may be discogenic, the Cyriax or McKenzie approach may be the first to be tried. However, if the evaluation reveals more of an apophyseal joint involvement and specific areas of dysfunction can be identified, the osteopathic or Paris approach may be indicated. The Maitland approach may be used if pain is the patient's primary complaint and it is difficult to correlate the subjective complaints with any structure or function. If the patient is exhibiting some chronic pain behavior, the evaluating practitioner may wish to deemphasize pain by emphasizing a mechanical evaluation of function.

The evaluation may indicate that the muscles are playing a primary role in pain production. Soft tissue massage techniques with spray and stretch could be indicated, sometimes in conjunction with joint mobilization techniques. The muscles, however, may not be painful, but may be causing altered stresses on the ligaments and joints of the spine preventing long-term improvement with joint mobilization. If a muscle is chronically tight, Janda's approach to stretching may be indicated. If the evaluation reveals muscle weakness and altered muscle firing patterns, the need for a strengthening program to the weakened musculature is indicated. If a tight muscle is not responding to stretch, deep connective tissue massage may be utilized to mechanically increase flexibility or reflexively allow the muscles to relax and respond to passive stretching.

It may become evident from the evaluation that certain patients do not wish to be touched, responding negatively to a direct mechanical approach. These patients may have had traumatic incidences such as a motor vehicle accident or previous negative experiences associated with touch. These patients most likely will get worse with direct manipulation or an aggressive exercise training program. Gentle, indirect hands-on treatment involving myofascial release, craniosacral therapy, or functional technique may be the first line of treatment for these patients. As their pain becomes better and they feel more comfortable with hands-on treatment, they can be progressed to a more direct approach. Limiting one's approach to only craniosacral therapy, myofascial release, or the indirect approach greatly limits the treating practitioner's ability to treat the whole patient. These approaches do not significantly change the patient's mechanical situation and may breed dependency on treatment while decreasing the effectiveness of the self-exercise program.

The evaluation of the chronic pain patient may reveal changes in coordination of the muscles in response to pain. These changes may be a significant perpetuating factor in the patient's chronic back pain due to the muscle's inability to properly support the ligaments and joints with activities of daily living. PNF, NDT, and working on proper muscle firing sequence would be indicated for this patient. Once the patient's joint function, muscle imbalances, and coordination have been addressed, the patient can be progressed to a general fitness program working on strength, endurance, and flexibility. The patient should receive individualized instruction to ensure that all the exercises are helpful and none accentuate the LBP. For instance, a patient with a symptomatic lytic spondylolisthesis that becomes aggravated with weight bearing, standing, and walking, would not be advised to start running, but would be encouraged to bike or do low impact aerobic activity. A patient with a herniated nucleus pulposis would be encouraged to perform activities that would avoid prolonged flexion with weight bearing. The patient should also be instructed in exercise activities that simulate the desired activity they are planning to resume. Once patients feel comfortable with their fitness program, they can be weaned completely from hands-on therapy and allowed to become independent with their rehabilitation program.

This has been a brief summary on the ideal clinical approach to patients with LBP. Patients with LBP are complex and it is difficult to be certain of the origin of their pain. It is important to reassess the patient frequently and be prepared to significantly change the course of treatment if the present course is not working. The length of treatment may last from one week to one year depending on the involvement of the patient. There are some other factors that depend less on actual treatment use, but can make a significant difference in the overall result of conservative treatment for LBP.

Open-Mindedness

Management of lower back pain is still in its infancy. Research demonstrates the effectiveness of surgery for some lumbar pathologies. Many patients with LBP do not have significant pathology that is evident on radiological imaging and, fortunately, most patients with LBP do not require surgery. These patients with nonspecific LBP are in need of conservative care for their problem. As indicated in the first part of this chapter, there are many types of conservative management available for patients with LBP. It is important for practitioners who provide conservative care for patients with LBP to seek out new types of treatment approaches, scrutinize them carefully, and integrate them into their overall approach.

Patient Management

Awareness of nonclinical factors in the treatment of LBP is an important aspect in the "perfect treatment." Communication is one factor that must not be overlooked. One must first listen carefully and empathetically to the patient. It seems that many patients are rushed through evaluations with overbooked medical providers who move them through the process so fast that the patients never are allowed to verbalize their specific pain complaints, let alone any other associated feelings or problems they are experiencing. Active listening by the physical therapist can provide valuable information regarding the clinical behavior of patients' pain. It also gives patients the message that the therapist is interested in them and wants to make them better. This can greatly enhance the first impression patients receive and allow for much better rapport between the therapist and patients. This kind of relationship encourages patients to become more cooperative with their home program.

After giving patients a chance to verbalize their concerns, it is important for the treating therapist to communicate what was found on the evaluation and what the course of treatment will be. The treatment plan should include some concrete, functional goals for the patient and the therapist to work on and allow both to assess whether the patient has improved. It is important to stress from the beginning of treatment that the long-term goal of treatment is patient self-management and independence from passive treatment for the back problem. If the patient knows this from the beginning, this will decrease the chance of the patient becoming dependent on physical therapy treatment and wanting to come in continuously for palliative treatment. If patients know their therapist's expectations initially, it will better allow them to work for the goal of independent treatment. This will benefit the patient both physically and psychologically and should decrease the overall cost of the treatment rendered.

The treating physical therapist should be aware of any psychological or social concerns associated with the patient's lower back problem. A patient who sees the treating therapist 2 to 3 times a week and has a good rapport with this therapist may verbalize concerns that the medical doctor, psychologist, or other treating practitioner who sees the patient less often is not aware of. The treating therapist should be aware of all the medical practitioners the patient is seeing and should know of some good psychologists, social workers, and chronic pain physicians if the patient requires these services.

Although physical therapy and physical management of LBP is a very important part of the patient's rehabilitation program, it is by no means the only approach. Therapists need to realize that they cannot effectively treat every patient alone and that working synergistically with other health care practitioners can benefit the patient much more in the long run.

Conclusion

Physical therapists today have many valuable tools to treat patients with LBP. This chapter has reviewed some of the clinical and nonclinical approaches to the treatment of patients with LBP. It appears the "perfect treatment" is an ideal practitioners should always try to attain. Development of the "perfect treatment" is an ongoing process. No matter what the clinical level of the physical therapist is, it is never too early to start. Therapists have the tools to treat patients with LBP the day they graduate from PT school. Therapists, however, should have a sincere desire to help the patient, believe that physical therapy can be effective in treating their patients, and desire to continue learning and refining their treatment approach, not taking it personally when a patient does not improve. By using the clinical tools they presently have, listening to the patient, and seeking out new treatment approaches through continuing education, research, and reading, all therapists can start developing their treatment approach today. With this attitude, the patient with a diagnosis of LBP can be an exciting challenge instead of the "problem" patient on the schedule. This attitude toward lower back patients will continue to improve the quality of conservative care for these patients and enhance the image of physical therapy as the profession that provides the most effective conservative care to patients who have LBP.

References

1. McKenzie RA: The Lumbar Spine: Mechanical Diagnosis and Therapy. New Zealand Spinal Publications Limited, 1981.
2. Williams PC: Evaluation and conservative treatment for disc lesions of the lower spine. Clin Orthop 5:28–40, 1955.
3. Mennell J: Back Pain Diagnosis and Treatment Using Manipulative Techniques. Boston, Little, Brown & Co., 1960.
4. Mennell J: Joint Pain Diagnosis and Treatment Using Manipulative Techniques. Boston, Little, Brown & Co., 1964.

5. Cyriax J: Textbook of Orthopedic Medicine, Vol 1, Diagnosis of Soft Tissue Lesions. London, Buelliere Tindall, 1978.

6. Nachemson A, Lind: In vivo measurements of intradiscal pressure. J Bone Joint Surg, 46A, 1077, 1975.

7. Stoddard A: Manual of Osteopathic Technique, 3rd ed. London, Hutchinson & Co., 1980.

8. Greenman PE: Principles of Manual Medicine. Baltimore, Williams and Wilkins, 1989.

9. Maitland GD: Vertebral Manipulation, 5th ed. Boston, MA, Butterworths 1986.

10. Donelson R, Silva G, Murphy K: Centralization phenomenon: Its usefulness in evaluating and treating referred pain. Spine 15:3 211–213, 1990.

11. Paris SV: The Paris approach. Post Graduate Advances in the Evaluation and Treatment of Low Back Dysfunction I–II. Forum Medicum Inc., 1989.

12. Paris SV: Component motions with special reference to the knee. Orthop Phys Ther 2(2), 1975.

13. Travell JG, Simons DG: Myofascial Pain and Dysfunction: The Trigger Point Manual. Baltimore, Williams and Wilkins, 1983.

14. Sahrmann S: Posture and muscle imbalance: Faulty lumbo-pelvic alignment and associated musculoskeletal pain syndromes. Post Graduate Advances in Physical Therapy, VIII APTA, 1987.

15. Kendall H, Kendall F, Boynton D: Posture and Pain. New York, Williams and Wilkins, 1952.

16. Janda V: Muscle Function Testing. London, Butterworths, 1983.

17. Lewitt K: Manipulative Therapy in Rehabilitation of the Motor System. London, Butterworths, 1985.

18. Sherrington C: The Integrative Action of the Nervous System. Hew Haven, CT, Yale University Press, 1947.

19. Voss D, Ionta M, Myers B: Proprioceptive Neuromuscular Facilitation: Patterns and Techniques, 3rd cd. Philadelphia, Harper and Row, 1985.

20. Bobath B: Adult Hemiplegia: Evaluation and Treatment, 2nd ed. London, William Clowes and Sons Limited, 1978.

21. Mitchell F, Moran P, Pruzzo N: An Evaluation and Treatment Manual of Osteopathic Muscle Energy Procedures. Valley Park, MO, 1979.

22. Jones LH: Strain and Counterstrain. Colorado Springs, CO, American Academy of Osteopathy, 1983.

23. Tappan F: Healing Massage Techniques: A Study of Eastern and Western Methods. Reston, VA, Prentice Hall Co.

24. Pruden B: Pain Erasure: The Bonnie Pruden Way. New York, Ballantine Books, 1980.

25. Mennell J: Physical Treatment by Movement Manipulation and Massage, 5th ed. Philadelphia, Blakston Co., and London, JA Churchill Limited, 1945.

26. Grodin A, Cantu R: Myofascial manipulation: Theory and clinical management. Post Graduate Advances in the Evaluation and Treatment of Low Back Dysfunction. Forum Medicine, 1989.
27. Upledger J, Vredevoogd J: Craniosacral Therapy. Seattle, WA, Eastland Press, 1984.
28. Magoun H. Osteopathy in the Cranial Field, 3rd ed. Kirksville, MO, Journal Printing Co., 1976.
29. Mayer T: Functional Restoration for Spinal Disorders: The Sports Medicine Approach. Philadelphia, Lea and Febiger, 1988.
30. Stratka SW, Newsome LS: The Use of Physical Modalities and Electrotherapy in the Treatment of Patients with Low Back Pain. Berryvill, VA, Forum Medicine Inc., 1–8, 1989.
31. Kellet K, Kellet D: Effects of an exercise program on sick leave. Phys Ther 71:4, 283–290, 1991.
32. Cady L, Bischoff D, O'Connell: Strength and fitness and subsequent back injuries in firefighters. J Occup Med 21:269–272, 1979.
33. Gunnari H, Evjenth O, Brady M: Sequence Exercise: The Sensible Approach to All-Around Fitness. Oslo, Dreyers Forlag, 1984.
34. Sale D: Neural adapation to resistance training. Medicine in Science and Sports and Exercise 2:5, 135–145, 1988.
35. Wyke B: The Lumbar Spine and Back Pain, 2nd ed. Ed by Jayson, London, Sector Publishing Limited, 265–340, 1976.
36. Finneson B: Low Back Pain, 2nd ed. Philadelphia, J. B. Lippincott Co., 179–197, 1980.
37. Sarno J: Healing Back Pain: The Mind Body Connection. New York, Warner Books, 1–97, 1991.

2

Exercise Prescription for Low Back Pain

Brian P. D'Orazio

Exercise is widely prescribed as a treatment for patients with low back pain (LBP). Excluding the use of medication and surgery, exercise is virtually the only scientifically validated form of treatment. Haldeman states, "There is now a convincing body of research that demonstrates that strengthening exercise together with improvement of cardiovascular fitness and general functional restoration can reduce disability and possibly pain in patients with chronic low back pain."[1] Research, however, is still extremely limited, with controlled studies being conducted on only a few specific exercise protocols.

While the quantity of published research using exercise as a treatment for LBP is inadequate, there are many successful empirical models of exercise that may be applicable. Most salient are the exercise programs used by bodybuilders, power lifters, and athletes in other sports which are dominated by strength training techniques. From these successful athletic programs and the existing exercise research on LBP, useful information can be extracted and applied to clinical situations.

The application of these empirical concepts into LBP programs need not be complex. One of the competitors in a women's bodybuilding contest several years ago had undergone two prior back surgeries. As described by the announcers for the competition, the surgeries had not been completely successful in eliminating her back pain; furthermore, other forms of treatment had been equally disappointing. The competitor embarked on a self-prescribed exercise program that gradually eased her pain, thus stimulating a greater desire for exercise. During the competition, there were no visible signs that this young woman had any prior back problems, as evidenced by her remarkable back flexibility and muscular definition.

This example of one person's success in overcoming chronic LBP contrasts with some authors' contentions that exercise is effective only when accompanied by an accurate diagnosis.[2] The improbability of an accurate diagnosis is best summarized in the 1987 monograph published in *Spine*, entitled "Scientific Approach to the Assessment and Management of Activity-Related Spinal Disorders."[3] In chapter three of this monograph the authors note, "It is generally impossible to corroborate clinical observations through histologic studies, because on one hand the usual benignity of spinal disorders does not justify that tissue be removed and, on the other, there is often no modification of tissue identifiable through current methods."

While an accurate diagnosis cannot be affixed to most LBP complaints, many exercise protocols purport to address specific pathologies. These theories of pathology typically focus on one tissue—with evaluation and management protocols so complex, the implementation of these theories could become a lifelong study. The psychosocial complexities of clinical interventions notwithstanding, exercise prescriptions for patients with LBP should borrow heavily from the basics of exercise and not become mired in complex theories meant to justify therapeutic interventions on patients without a diagnosis.

Definitions

There are several key words that deserve special consideration. The first and most important is *strength*. Strength, in the context of this chapter, describes the ability to generate a maximum amount of force through a range of motion or at any given point in that range. The second term, *endurance*, describes the ability of an individual to repeat a task over a period of time. Finally, *flexibility* describes a system of tissues that allows a joint to move through a range of motion. Flexibility in this context does not describe the extensibility of a specific tissue.

In this chapter's literature review, each author's use of these terms is interpreted as it applies to the research question. Hopefully, this will reduce confusion; however, those reading this chapter may find their interpretation of the literature differs, based in part on the lack of definition for these terms in published research.

Where Did We Begin?

Many twentieth century theories on exercise prescription for LBP can be traced to the two-part series published in 1937 by Paul C. Williams, entitled, "Lesions of the Lumbosacral Spine."[4,5] The articles, probably read by few clinicians practicing today, were an ambitious undertaking by Williams who reported his findings were based on a study of 1,000 chronic LBP cases. The tenets of the articles were promptly accepted by the medical field and soon were embraced by the general population. Remarkably, the articles are almost purely anecdotal and offer virtually no statistical support for any observations. Nevertheless, the articles have had a profound influence on the care of LBP patients.

Williams, during a time of evolving interest in the intervertebral disc, was convinced that LBP was the result of pathological lumbar intervertebral discs. He believed this pathology was the result of humankind's lumbar lordosis. Accentuating the compressive traumatic forces to the posterior aspect of the intervertebral disc, the lumbar lordosis ultimately led to encroachment of nerve roots, he reported. Historically, Williams stated, most lifting accidents could be traced to the position in which "the patient had lifted the load to such a height that the lumbosacral lordosis was restored." This interesting view of the injury mechanism supported Williams' belief that the lumbar erector spinae were overdeveloped "at the expense of the antagonistic flexor muscles." He felt this "imbalance" in the lumbar spine resulted in a lumbar lordosis. Therefore, he viewed the lordosis "as a pathological deformity" despite his recognition that the lordosis was common. Williams' therapeutic interventions, whether conservative or surgical, were consequently designed to eliminate the cause of LBP; namely, the lordosis. He even went so far as to state, "It will be noted that the principles herein outlined are directed toward the restoration of those muscles which are sacrificed by the erect posture, and the restoration of the contour of the lower spine to resemble as nearly as possible that of the quadruped animal."[5] The theory that mankind had perhaps not fully or properly evolved, thereby explaining our vulnerability to LBP, likely originated from this belief.

The general principles of treatment, as outlined by Williams, were applied for acute and chronic pain essentially despite his physical findings. Initially the patient was placed in a plaster cast and forward flexed enough to completely eradicate the lumbosacral lordosis. Most patients were then placed on bed rest for ten days or possibly longer, depending on their relief from symptoms. After this time, the patient was permitted to ambulate with the plaster cast for an additional one to two weeks based on symptoms. Upon removal of the cast, the patient was placed in a back brace intended to maintain the flattened lumbar lordosis. This brace was worn for three to twelve months, depending primarily on the patient's age. Once the patient was essentially free from symptoms, postural exercises were initiated which became known as *Williams' flexion exercises*. This series, well-known to most clinicians, was intended to reinforce the concept of maintaining a flattened lordosis while restoring a proper balance between spinal flexors and extensors. The contribution of muscle imbalance to LBP is a common theme brought forward in some contemporary theories on causes of back pain. The four original exercises, shown in Figure 2.1, lacked parameters for their performance.

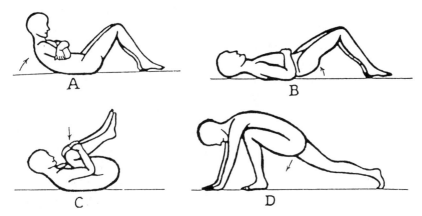

Figure 2.1 Postural exercises designed to reduce the lumbosacral angle: (A) active development of the abdominal muscles; (B) active development of the gluteal and hamstring muscles; (C) passive stretching of the sacrospinalis; (D) passive stretching of the hip flexors. (Reprinted with permission from Tilton S, Williams PC: Lesions of the Lumbosacral Spine. Part 2. JBJS 19:699, 1937.)

Reviewing the Williams' articles demonstrates how easily anecdotal information can influence clinical practice. The remarkable number of theories in these articles is based singularly on the intervertebral disc as the cause of symptoms with the lumbar lordosis as the primary cause of disc pathology. Many of these theories are memorable even from my childhood, when my first-grade teacher examined our posture by having us stand against the wall. She indicated to us that she should not be able to pass her hand between the wall and our back. If she was able to do so, we were considered to have "bad posture." Corroborating this personal experience, Williams stated "certain expressions such as 'sit up straight,' 'throw your chest out,' and 'draw in your abdomen' should be stricken from our postural programs." Williams taught that proper lifting technique involved maintaining a pelvic tilt while lifting with our legs. Further, he felt that to have the correct sitting posture one must sit with the hips slightly below the knees and "sit in a slightly slumped position. . . ." Williams felt that chair design should eliminate the lumbosacral lordosis, thus avoiding LBP. Interestingly, Williams ended his two-part series by stating, "It has been the writer's experience that a well planned [sic] conservative program will eliminate the need for surgery in most cases." The failure of Williams' "well-planned conservative program" constituted a reason to perform surgery.

As it was Williams' belief that surgery should be performed after the failure of a prolonged conservative program, his articles also imply that he achieved excellent clinical results with conservative treatment. In one of the few statistics that Williams shares, he reported performing surgery on only thirty-six patients in a subgrouping of four hundred patients. Only twenty of these surgeries were reported to be purely disc-related. The implication is that the 364 chronic LBP patients who did not have surgery were either cured or significantly improved as a result of conservative care. This statistic defies current research regarding results from treatment of chronic LBP patients regardless of the method employed.

Williams' approach to treatment and his beliefs regarding causes of LBP have to be disregarded in their entirety based on the lack of statistical support for his conclusions. Further, his conservative program is barbaric by today's standards. The question to be posed is whether Williams' patients improved because of or in spite of his intervention. Clinicians should become familiar with these articles as they have had a dramatic impact on clinical care.

In one of few studies directly challenging the use of Williams' flexion exercises, Ponte et al.[6] demonstrated, in a small sample, that the protocol developed by McKenzie produced better results in a shorter time than Williams' flexion exercises. While the sample was small, it is interesting to note that the authors described improvement in both treatment groups, despite antagonistic theories and essentially antagonistic exercise programs. The exercises advocated by Williams, however, were intended to be used only at the end of a long course of treatment that included bed rest, casting, and bracing. The comparison between the two protocols, therefore, is out of context with Williams' articles but is relevant to the contemporary use of Williams' program.

The Williams articles and the article by Ponte et al. demonstrate the need to closely scrutinize theories on back pain and back pain management. The rigid application of anecdotal information to patient care is destructive when it extinguishes the use of existing research to guide clinical decisions. Many current theories on the origins of back pain are similarly based on anecdotal information that is unsubstantiated by existing research. Consequently, the next section of this chapter will review research and contemporary views on exercise as a treatment for LBP.

What Do We Know about LBP Exercise Programs?

In 1955, Flint was one of the first to report progressive resistive exercises being prescribed for patients with LBP.[7] In this study, 19 females described as having chronic LBP were placed on a treatment program consisting only of exercise, three times each week. Resistance was applied throughout the patient's full available range in both flexion and extension. Ten repetitions of each exercise were performed followed by ten additional sit-ups against resistance. A control group of 27 women was taken through the same program. Flint reported significant gains in strength for flexion and extension in both groups. Symptoms completely resolved in eleven patients and partially resolved in six. Five of the six patients who experienced partial relief did not complete their programs. Of the two subjects who reported no relief of symptoms, one was irregular in attendance and the other was released because of increased pain following exercises. Despite Flint's findings, there seems to be no direct follow-up in the literature regarding the effects of progressive resistive exercises on LBP. In fact, the number of studies performed on exercise related to LBP is very small.

The Quebec Task Force on Spinal Disorders reported that exercise, whether performed in a specialized center or at home, was commonly prescribed but lacked a body of scientific evidence to support its use prior to seven weeks after an injury.[3] After this time, the Task Force's findings indicate reasonable support in the literature to substantiate its usefulness. Studies used in the report, such as those by Davies et al.[8] and Kendall and Jenkins,[9] present with equivocal findings that were likely viewed by the Task Force to not strongly support the use of exercise for LBP treatment.

A more recent work lending support to the concept that exercise is beneficial in subacute patients was published in 1990 by Mitchell and Carmen.[10] Their study compared 951 patients with work-related injuries who were treated at twelve clinics using specified guidelines to 2,172 matched subjects treated at other centers using a variety of methods. All subjects were referred no more than 10 weeks and not less than 22 days after their injury. The twelve clinics used a three-phase protocol of treatment including: (1) pain relief and mobilization; (2) increased movement and muscle strengthening; (3) further strengthening and work conditioning. The exercise portion of the program was characterized by the following description: "General body fitness, strength, and endurance were the main components of work conditioning achieved by the sequence training equipment and the cardiovascular fitness machines. . . . There was little emphasis placed on work simulation, although a lift station was a component of the gymnasium." The primary criterion delineating results from the twelve clinics and the matched group was the cost of compensable benefits. This included heath care costs as well as wage loss costs. When proportionately adjusted, compensation costs were $5,584,109 for the experimental group compared to $7,155,076 for the control group. Days lost from work were 88,404 in the experimental group and 127,611 in the comparison group. This study demonstrates that exercise has a positive therapeutic value, even in subacute patients where the natural progression of LBP was previously thought to account for virtually all improvement.

The Task Force also did not appear to review the 1981 study of Fordyce, who examined the relationship between complaints of pain and exercise performance in patients with chronic LBP.[11] In the twenty-five retrospective cases studied, these authors concluded, "These data indicate that, at least for the chronic pain patients studied here, the more exercises performed, the fewer the pain complaints or visible/audible expression of pain." The 1985 research by Mayer et al. is one of the first comprehensive studies to incorporate a graded exercise program into an overall rehabilitation program for chronic LBP patients.[12] Their study, while compelling, involved multiple disciplines treating the patient's physical dysfunction as well as addressing sociological and psychological issues. The contribution of exercise, therefore, cannot be specifically extracted from this study.

Is Trunk Strength an Important Variable of Low Back Pain?

The cause-effect relationship between trunk strength and low back pain remains a controversial issue. Virtually all studies support the concept that trunk strength is reduced among patients with chronic LBP.[12-17] The studies also indicate that cardiovascular fitness is compromised and trunk extensor endurance is diminished among chronic LBP patients.[18-20] From industrial studies it is well accepted that heavier jobs are associated with an increased incidence of LBP.[21-23] Other studies have indicated that greater trunk strength is not likely to prevent LBP[24] and has little prognostic value to indicate who is likely to develop LBP.[19] None of these studies, however, have extensively examined the cause-effect relationship between preinjury strength and current symptoms.

In a longitudinal study, Leino et al. studied 902 employees in a metal industry, investigating the cause and effect relationships between back pain and trunk strength.[25] Of the original 902 employees, 654 were reexamined after 10 years. The study concluded, "The subjects with clinical findings in the low back at the baseline had worse results in the muscle function tests at the follow up than the subjects with normal backs; the results of those with the most findings were the worst." Their conclusion was that decreased force production resulted from chronic clinical findings and in many cases, caused symptoms.

Despite the paucity of research and some conflicting reports, the preponderant evidence indicates that decreased back strength contributes to chronicity among LBP patients and is a significant variable contributing to the pain formula when individuals are mismatched for their activity. That is to say, individuals undertaking heavy lifting tasks are more likely to injure themselves if their trunk strength is inadequate.

Rehabilitation Theories for Low Back Pain

Given the scant research available on LBP exercises, it is reasonable to conclude there are no widely accepted contemporary exercise models for patients with LBP. Examining the more popular exercise strategies and their respective working diagnoses can be helpful in developing a rationale for exercise prescription.

Stabilization Exercises

Lumbar instability, while heavily researched, is difficult to define clinically. Manually, the technique of passive intersegmental mobility testing (PIMT) has been examined in two studies. The research by Gonnella, Paris, and Kutner examined intratester and intertester reliability in PIMT of the lumbar spine.[26] The presentation of data and statistical analysis, however, is seriously flawed, rendering the study inconclusive. The study by Kaltenborn and Lindahl presents better data in support of PIMT; however, instability is never demonstrated to be a clinical problem and, as with the Gonnella study, validity cannot be inferred based on their reports of reliability.[27] Neither can it be assumed that the skill required to reliably perform PIMT is uniformly present among all clinicians using PIMT.

The radiographic literature is similarly confusing. Some authors assume that if hypertrophic changes are noted, hypermobility must exist.[28] The anatomical study by Gertzbein et al. does not completely support this assumption.[29] Gertzbein's research demonstrated the greatest evidence for instability was in discs with little or no radiographic evidence of degeneration. Further, they noted, in degenerative discs "the major abnormality of motion is erratic rather than excessive movement." The fact that radiography is known to underestimate degenerative changes[30] and consistently fails to discriminate between subjects with and without LBP[31] should cause skepticism when reviewing radiographic information used to identify benign lumbar instability or hypermobility.

Despite the controversy, dynamic lumbar stabilization techniques are gaining popularity in the treatment of LBP. This exercise philosophy promotes maintenance of a neutral, pain-free position between the lumbar spine and pelvis.[2] The neutral position is maintained primarily through contraction of the abdominal musculature. Once patients learn to maintain this neutral position during normal postures, they are taught to lift while maintaining this position. Patients then apply these principles to a total rehabilitation program including riding a stationary bike, running on a treadmill, swimming, weight lifting and other exercises. The intent is to minimize stress on the lumbar spine and stabilize unstable motion segments. Saal and Saal in describing rehabilitation of back pain patients using dynamic stabilization techniques state, "Obviously a patient in severe pain inadequately controlled by the principles set forth in this chapter should undergo the appropriate surgical procedure earlier than the suggested three month time period."[2] Again, the decision regarding surgery is based, in large measure, on the success of the exercise program. It is difficult to determine whether the decision to perform surgery in these cases is based on the philosophy that instability is the cause of the patient's pain or whether there is some other clinical justification for the surgery. There is, as yet, no published research on dynamic lumbar stabilization. Its underlying premise of stabilizing motion segments is questionable.

McKenzie's Theory of Exercise

McKenzie's techniques deserve attention, because of both their widespread use and their demonstrated value in patient care. McKenzie's program is detailed in chapter 1.

Postural Exercise

The role of altering posture to reduce back pain undoubtedly predates even the Williams' articles. Many theories on the subject have been popularized over the years, despite the paucity of scientific information defining proper posture or its relationship to back pain. The postural abnormality receiving the greatest clinical attention in benign cases of LBP is an increased lumbar lordosis. While there are no studies that quantitatively define an increased lordosis, much clinical dogma advocates strengthening the abdominal muscles or lengthening the lumbar erector spinae to reduce the lumbar curve. The ability of the abdominal muscles to alter the lumbar curve, however, has been questioned in a study by Walker et al., demonstrating that abdominal muscle performance in healthy subjects did not correlate to measures of lumbar lordosis or pelvic tilt.[32] On the contrary, they raised the question of whether muscular strength can determine the static position of a joint. Given the anatomical variance in the lumbar spine and pelvis, it seems unlikely that minor variations in posture between patients would cause symptoms.

Weight Training

With an increasing emphasis on objective results, an array of equipment has been developed to assist clinicians in substantiating claims of improvement. For the trunk, dynamometers are the most recent and promising tool toward that end. An old tool, however, is simply the lifting of a weight.

The activity of lifting a weight is objective in that increases can be easily documented. Despite limited research related to treatment of LBP, weight training has been gaining popularity as part of the *sports medicine approach* to treatment. The principles of weight training have a great empirical data base as evidenced by bodybuilding and power lifting competitions, wrestling, football, or any sport traditionally regarded as a strength sport. Application of these techniques to patients with LBP needs to be extensively studied but does show great promise.

The Use of Movement to Guide Exercise Prescription

Movement, whether purposeful or nonpurposeful, gross or fine, passive or active, is the common denominator to all therapeutic exercise interventions. Physical evaluations assess movements, then correlate movements with reports of pain in an attempt to diagnose the problem. Assumptions about the evaluation, such as the patient demonstrates his full capabilities, pain accurately reflects the patient's pathology, muscles always function synchronously to control movement, etc., are not always correct. For example, the problem created by symptom magnification is readily appreciated when attempting to prescribe treatment, as pain is often an inaccurate reflection of pathology. Equally inaccurate is the view that all abnormal movement patterns are the result of joint mechanical dysfunction. For this view to be valid, the given imperative would be that an individual's choice of movement pattern is predetermined by spinal mechanics.

Both the lack of diagnostic value in the patient's pain report and our current inability to relate movement and pathology create a dilemma in clinical examination. On the one hand, presumptions that are scientifically unvalidated may lead to erroneous conclusions; on the other hand, relying on what is known may render us incapable of performing a clinically useful examination. If, however, the issue of pathology is discarded for the moment, it may be possible to determine how movement is involved in the patient's pain complaint. The value of this determination, given that most of the time a definitive diagnosis is not possible, lies in the *prescription of treatment.* We must ardently pursue answers to the dilemma of diagnosis, but we should pursue meaningful treatment with the same ardor. The two are not mutually exclusive, and perhaps it will be through successful treatment regimes that meaningful diagnostic classifications are achieved.

In an attempt to move in a direction that defines segments of an examination that can produce meaningful exercise prescriptions, patterns of movement are divided into two types—static dysfunction (morphologic) and dynamic dysfunction (neuromuscular). The nomenclature signifies two distinct classifications of movement that are identifiable in patients with back pain. Typically, one of these movement types predominates. The following descriptions of these movement types are qualitative. Nevertheless, there are consistent, identifiable patterns in most patients that allow the clinician to differentiate one type from the other. Keep in mind that this is not another subtle attempt at diagnosing the problem. A specific pathologic diagnosis is not possible. Rather, these movement patterns should be viewed only as an indicator of treatment prescription.

Static Dysfunction

Static dysfunctions are defined as being the result of soft tissue restrictions and/or muscular atrophy. These commonly result from chronic pain but may also preexist the onset of pain. Chronic LBP patients, as noted previously, have been demonstrated to produce less trunk force and possess a decreased capacity to perform work. In my clinical experience, even when pain is no longer a factor, force production and endurance will remain below normal without a reconditioning program. Superimposed on iatrogenic changes secondary to chronic LBP are those changes that occurred prior to the patient developing LBP. An example is the hip flexor inflexibility commonly noted with truck drivers or those in occupations requiring prolonged sitting. Changes are also evident in some people who exercise repetitively. For example, long distance runners often develop inflexibility through the hip external rotators and back extensors. Static changes can also occur following disease or surgery.

Patients with predominantly static dysfunctions typically move near the end of their available range before experiencing significant pain. Their movement pattern, even if slightly guarded, is fairly well coordinated. These patients may forward bend only to the midtibial region; however, they are able to achieve that range before encountering great difficulty and they are then able to reassume an erect posture with minimal substitutive patterns. On further examination, the reason for the restricted motion is often clear; that is, some structure such as the hamstrings or back extensors are inflexible independent from the pain response.

Dynamic Dysfunction

Patients with dynamic dysfunction have difficulty coordinating simple movements. For example, standing forward bending utilizes more than sagittal plane motion, and reassuming an erect posture often requires assistance. Frequently, patients are unable to move through even limited ranges without pain and typically cannot reach below their knees. Some clinicians may feel the symptoms are so severe that treatment cannot be instituted. Patients in this category can be acute or chronic. An examination reveals passive restrictions of motion are not nearly as limited as the patient's active mobility, thus demonstrating the potential for much greater range.

Most patients in this "dynamic" category indicate they would be able to move through greater ranges but are limited by pain. Rather, it is the dynamic dysfunction often causing continuing symptoms. This is best demonstrated by those patients who initially present with virtually no movement and are then able, after a hands-off movement guided program, to forward bend and palm the floor, lift small weights, and subsequently leave the office reporting much less discomfort. It is important to recognize pain as a symptom of dysfunction, not necessarily reflecting the severity of the pathology. For example, a cramp in the ankle plantar flexors is most certainly a painful phenomenon, but it is rare that the cramp itself is serious.

Patients with dynamic dysfunction present with varied histories. Some have received substantial trauma; others are unable to stand up after bending over to tie their shoes. Sometimes the pain is of immediate onset or symptoms can occur slowly, as with the patient who presents with pain 24 to 48 hours following an automobile accident.

Combined Dysfunctions

Almost always, patients present with a combination of these two dysfunctions. Probably one predominates, but therapeutically, if the patient's condition contains a dynamic component, that dysfunction is best addressed prior to treating the static dysfunction. Typically, the dynamic dysfunction can be resolved quickly, within the first one to five visits, at which time a better appreciation is gained for the amount of static involvement.

Viewing dysfunction in this manner does not alter any eventual hypothesis regarding a diagnosis, nor does it infringe on any specific philosophies such as osteopathic, McKenzie, Paris, or others. Rather, it organizes the clinical approach, allowing the clinician to make reasonable judgments about the type of therapeutic exercise intervention to be used and how treatment should be sequenced. For example, patients generally should not enter a progressive resistive exercise program if the dynamic component to their problem has not substantially resolved. The addition of extra resistance will likely result in further aberrations of motion with reports of increased discomfort.

By combining observations of movements with what is suspected regarding pathology (For example, there is a continuing inflammatory process or the patient is experiencing muscle spasm that is creating the movement dysfunction), the clinician may make other reasonable choices about therapeutic interventions. For example, the patient with primarily a static problem who arises in the morning without as much discomfort as he experiences later in the day probably does not have a significant inflammatory process associated with that dysfunction.

Dynamic Exercise Prescription

A successful dynamic exercise program is contingent on the patience and persistence of both clinician and patient. There are many ways to resolve the dynamic dysfunction. The following describes the method I have developed.

Prior to entering this phase of rehabilitation, patients should comprehend why they have pain and why they are unable to move. I like to use the analogy of having a cramp. I explain that a cramp in the calf is a fairly simple phenomenon. As such, an individual can instinctively determine how to eliminate the cramp, thus gaining relief. After the cramp has been relieved, the muscle remains irritable, subjecting it to a repeated cramp if movements are uncontrolled. If a second cramp occurs, stretching will rapidly alleviate symptoms. The back, on the other hand, is a far more complex structure. Consequently, there is no innate sense of how to alleviate the spasm. Patients are told that the exercises prescribed are patterned movements, intended to relieve the spasm and subsequently to relieve discomfort. It is essential they understand the pain cannot be eliminated prior to normalizing function. This explanation should be delivered within the context of the patient's condition. As an example, I treated a patient who injured herself when she bent forward to perform a task at work and then was unable to reassume an erect posture. During the course of interviewing this patient, it became clear that she needed a very direct understandable explanation for her continuing dilemma. During the examination, there were two audible manipulations following which the patient reported a slight decrease in discomfort and she was able to move slightly better than before. The changes in her function were relatively insignificant; however, an explanation that the joints may have become "stuck" seemed to alleviate anxiety regarding her condition. I was then able to proceed with the explanation that remaining spasm would be eliminated with a dynamic movement program. By the end of the session, the patient was able to forward bend and touch the floor without discomfort. The point is, regardless of the clinician's or the patient's opinions regarding the cause of their problem, the patient needs to be offered a plausible explanation for why they must be put through such a rigorous program to regain control of function.

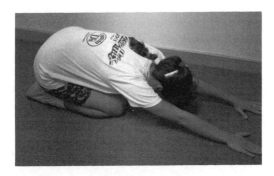

Figure 2.2 Full quadruped flexion.

Once patients understand the nature of their problem, depending on the physical examination, I begin having them perform repeated, pain-free, quadruped flexions (Figure 2.2). During the *first* series of between 15 and 20 repetitions, the patient is encouraged to move in pain-free ranges, gradually attempting greater movements. Some patients are willing to move through greater ranges, while others need assistance. Assistance is provided by hands-on guidance which should not be perceived as forcing movement.

Repetitive seated flexion (Figure 2.3) is the next exercise. This eventually should be performed by having the patient slide his hands down the lateral aspect of his legs in pain-free ranges. Initially, the patient may need to perform this movement by pushing off the knees to reduce active use of the extensors, thereby controlling symptoms. Some patients have an easier time with seated flexion than with quadruped flexion while for others the reverse is true. Seated flexion is also repeated 15 to 20 times. I often leave the patient's room to allow some independence in this activity.

The next phase is based on the quality of movement. When both quadruped flexion and seated flexion are through nearly full ranges, the patient

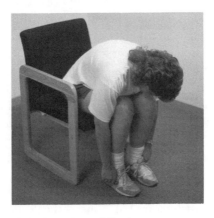

Figure 2.3 Seated flexion.

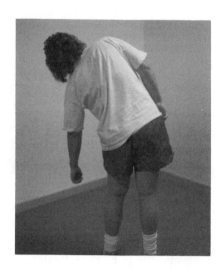

Figure 2.4 Standing lateral trunk bends.

progresses to 15 to 20 repetitions of standing lateral bends through pain-free ranges (Figure 2.4). If quadruped or seated flexion remains limited, these movements are repeated, sometimes encouraging the patient to move into slightly painful ranges. If nearly full ranges of motion are not achieved, the patient will perform only those two movements for the remainder of that session and no further movements will be given for the patient's home program.

It is common for patients to experience extreme fatigue from these exercises. Patients should be reassured that the fatigue they are experiencing will reduce dramatically once the movements are well coordinated. It is important to persist in teaching patients these movements either until physical activity can no longer be tolerated or until they are able to move successfully through nearly full ranges of motion.

The next phase is repetitive forward and backward bending while standing (Figure 2.5). Patients are instructed to move through pain-free ranges while keeping their hands in contact with their legs. Initially, I limit forward bending so the patients' hands do not move past their knees. This avoids having patients unexpectedly move into a painful range from which they may be unable to reassume an erect posture. If this occurs, assist the patient in reassuming an erect posture. Quadruped flexions should then be reinstituted and all phases repeated. If standing flexion and extension are progressing as expected, encourage the patient to gradually move through greater ranges until full range is achieved. The patient should be allowed to slightly flex his knees with this activity.

Quadruped flexion and *extension* is initiated if the previous phases are successfully completed (Figure 2.6). This activity will replace quadruped flexion while the other movements will remain the same. After one addi-

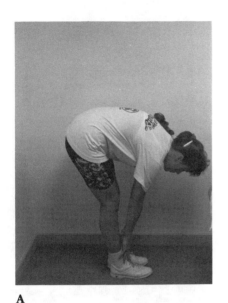

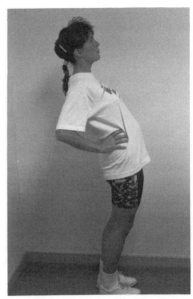

A   **B**

Figure 2.5 (A) Standing forward bending. (B) Standing backward bending.

tional set of each exercise, the patient should be able to move through full ranges with limited discomfort. Sometimes multiple sets, requiring 90 minutes or more, are necessary to achieve the desired end result of controlled movement.

If the patient rapidly moves through the entire program and achieves full ranges, standing lateral bends and standing flexion and extension can be progressed by using a light weight (Figures 2.7 and 2.8). In forward bending, the patient holds the dumbbell perpendicular to the floor, maintaining the knees

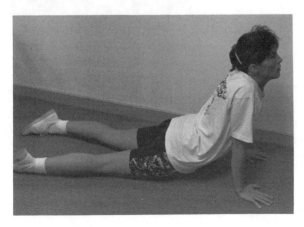

Figure 2.6 Quadruped extension.

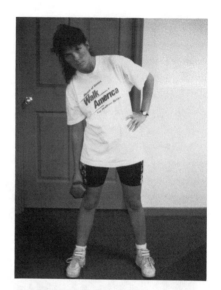

Figure 2.7 Resisted lateral trunk bends.

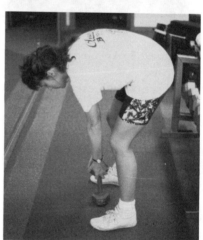

Figure 2.8 Vertical dumbbell dead lifts.

in a slightly flexed position. I usually start with no more than 5 pounds. By holding the weight perpendicular, the distance traveled is slightly less than what the patient had achieved without the weight. If the patient is successful in touching the weight to the floor, I have the patient hold the weight horizontally (Figure 2.9) and encourage greater motion.

The home exercise prescription is vitally important. Exercises must be performed at least hourly, in sets of 15 to 20 repetitions for every exercise. Standing flexion and extension is sometimes limited to only 10 repetitions per set if excessive fatigue through the back extensors is a problem. Patients are instructed not to panic if the "cramp" should recur. Rather, they should

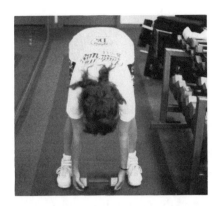

Figure 2.9 Horizontal dumbbell dead lifts.

immediately resume quadruped flexions and, once these have been performed successfully, their program should continue as during their first treatment session. The first home session must begin as soon as the patient returns home. Patients should be informed that they will likely feel "stiff" after getting out of the car following a 10-minute ride. For many patients, the entire series of exercises is repeated every 30 minutes for 6 hours before progressing to hourly sessions.

Whether the patient achieves control of motion in the first or fifth visit, it is evident that as control is gained, the patient's confidence improves and compliance with a home program is facilitated. In those few individuals who do not achieve success with the program, I will usually eliminate the dynamic exercises, use pain modalities, reassess my original hypothesis and possibly return to the dynamic exercise prescription within the next several visits.

Some patients seen during the acute phase may have little static involvement. Often, once normal control of motion has been restored, a patient may feel ready to resume normal activities. The patient should be taken through a brief functional assessment to make sure that lifting heavy objects does not provoke symptoms. Testing should be specific for the types of activities the patient is likely to encounter. If symptoms occur, I begin the patient on the static phase of the program.

I have detailed this aspect of the program primarily to highlight the decision-making process and the importance of follow through. There are many techniques to achieve dynamic neuromuscular control. I use this approach because the movements are basic, easily mastered, and relatively easy to regulate. For purposes of sequencing, the dynamic exercises are basic gross motor skills that I believe should precede fine motor coordination exercises. Isolated pelvic movements are difficult for patients who have discomfort and poor gross motor control. Expecting the patient to master fine motor skills at this stage will only frustrate the patient and the clinician.

Even if the clinician is strongly biased toward a specific diagnosis, this program is still usable in helping the patient redevelop gross motor skills. The most important point is that if neuromuscular coordination is impaired, movement in some form is at least part of the solution to the patient's problem.

Static Exercise Prescription

The static phase of a patient's program begins after he or she has reestablished good neuromuscular coordination. The primary deficit in motion should be related to iatrogenic changes. If the primary problem was dynamic, usually the pain level has reduced and the patient is confident that you will be able to help them achieve further improvements. If the dynamic portion of the problem was small in comparison to the overall problem, the patients' symptoms likely have changed very little. In any case, the clinician will have been given more information regarding the patient's chief problem.

Flexibility

If flexibility could not adequately be examined during the earlier visits, a full flexibility examination should now be performed. Correlations between the patient's chief complaint and areas of trunk or lower extremity inflexibility should be the starting point for a flexibility program. Because stretching involves time and a great deal of attention to symptoms, flexibility exercise prescriptions should be limited to only three or four stretches.

Most patients, even with extensive instructions, have difficulty grasping both the intent of the exercise and the intensity that should be attained during stretching. Typically, patients stretch too far, exacerbating symptoms. Patients should be informed that overstretching will likely occur, despite multiple cautions directed against such an effort. If they overstretch, patients are instructed to continue stretching as prescribed, decreasing intensity but not frequency. They should discontinue the exercise if they are uncertain how to proceed and have not been able to recontact the clinician for clarification.

Unfortunately, as with many exercises, there is no consensus regarding the proper performance of a stretch. I find that effective stretching is facilitated by relaxation. Patients should therefore be instructed to schedule a quiet time for stretching, allowing them to concentrate on relaxing. Ten to 20 seconds of each stretch is used to concentrate on relaxing the desired areas. Consequently, the patient is instructed to hold a stretched position for 40

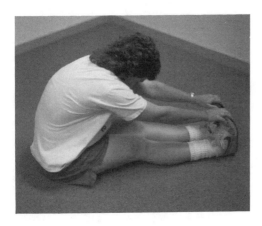

Figure 2.10 Long sitting stretch.

seconds. Usually, the stretch is alternated with the contralateral side; or, the patient is instructed to wait 15 seconds between stretches. Each stretch is repeated three to four times per session, allowing the patient to stretch at least once after experiencing some improvement in flexibility.

The nomenclature used to identify specific stretches in the next section is purely descriptive. The positions used are a result of both clinical and personal trial and error. Consequently, the nomenclature will not necessarily correspond to that described by other authors. The suggestions made in the following section represent only one way of accomplishing clinical goals.

Back Extensors

The central fibers of the back extensors can be stretched in multiple positions. The position that often provides the best stretch is *long sitting* (Figure 2.10). This position can be regulated by altering the amount of knee flexion based on flexibility through the hamstrings and what the patient is feeling while stretching. Other positions that may be of benefit include the *squat* position (Figure 2.11), the *fully-flexed quadruped* position (Figure 2.12), or sometimes the supine *knees to chest* position (Figure 2.13). Only the position providing the optimal stretch should be prescribed. Later in the program, this may change based on the patient's improvement.

The lateral fibers of the back extensors are usually best stretched in the *half-split* position (Figure 2.14). The area to be stretched is regulated principally by the position of the extended lower extremity. Abducting the extended lower extremity focuses the stretch more laterally. The patient's extended lower extremity may need to be slightly flexed at the knee to reduce tension in the hamstrings. Other positions which stretch the lateral fibers

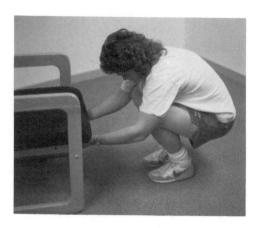

Figure 2.11 Squat stretch.

include the *seated lateral bending/rotation* stretch (Figure 2.15) or the *standing lateral bending* stretch (Figure 2.16) which also stretches the latissimus dorsi and the obliques.

Back Flexors

Abdominal contractures are found in some individuals who have had abdominal surgery and sometimes in runners. Stretching the rectus abdominis is performed as in Figure 2.17. While patients perform this stretch, which elevates the ribs and anteriorly tilts the pelvis, they are instructed to gently distend the abdomen, if needed, to provide additional stretching.

The iliopsoas is more commonly involved than are the abdominals. This muscle group can be stretched in several positions but usually is best stretched as demonstrated in Figure 2.18. In this position, the patient is encouraged to maintain a fully extended knee through the weightbearing

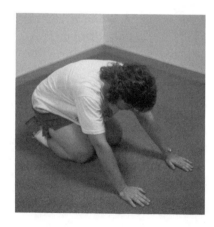

Figure 2.12 Fully flexed quadruped stretch.

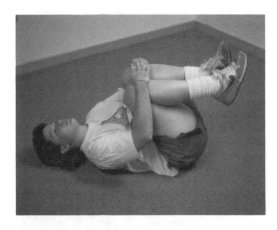

Figure 2.13 Supine knees to chest stretch.

limb while maintaining the lumbar spine in a neutral or slightly flexed position to control the intensity of stretching. The supine iliopsoas stretch is used when the patient is more involved. In these most involved patients, the extended lower extremity should remain supported on the table (Figure 2.19) prior to progressing to the unsupported position (Figure 2.20). The intensity of the stretch is regulated by the amount of flexion in the contralateral hip.

Hip External Rotators

The hip external rotators are commonly involved, often producing the patient's chief complaint of LBP. This is an extremely sensitive region that I find to be inflexible in most patients. There are multiple stretches for this region, some of which are depicted in Figures 2.21 and 2.22.

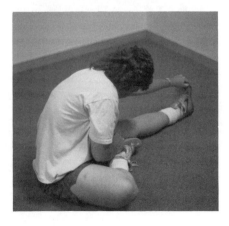

Figure 2.14 Half split stretch.

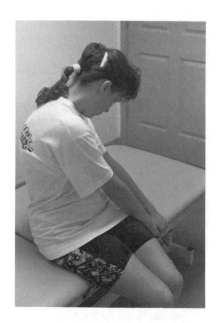

Figure 2.15 Seated lateral bending/ rotation stretch.

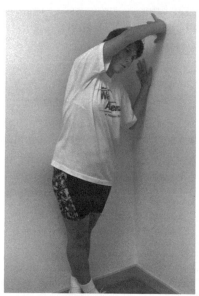

Figure 2.16 Standing lateral bending stretch.

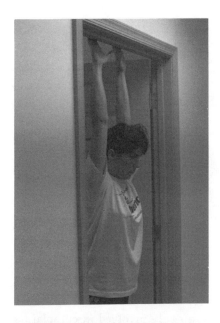

Figure 2.17 Rectus abdominis stretch.

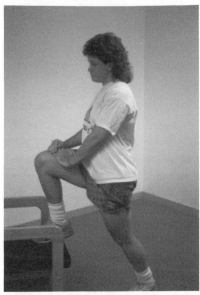

Figure 2.18 Standing iliopsoas stretch.

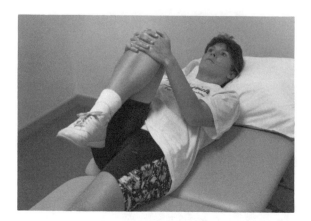

Figure 2.19 Supine iliopsoas stretch, supported.

Hip Abductors

The hip abductors are also commonly involved in complaints
of LBP. The Ober test position can be used to stretch the involved region;
however, this requires the clinician's intervention. Several stretch positions
can be performed without the clinician's intervention and these are depicted
in Figures 2.23, 2.24 and 2.25. If the abductors are extensively involved, two
of these positions may be necessary.

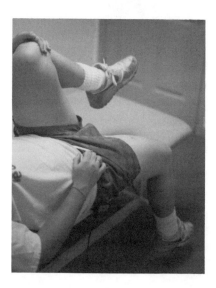

Figure 2.20 Supine iliopsoas stretch,
unsupported.

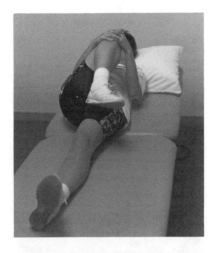

Figure 2.21 Hip external rotators stretch.

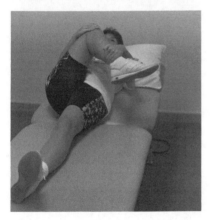

Figure 2.22 Hip external rotators stretch.

Hip Extensors

Hip extensor stretching is well understood by most clinicians. Any of the positions used to stretch the iliopsoas can be used to stretch the hip extensors in addition to positions such as the *squat* stretch and bilateral *knees to chest*.

Hamstrings

The hamstrings are stretched in a myriad of positions, with the most common complicating factors being either nerve root tension or inflexibility through the popliteal region. Allowing the foot and ankle to remain

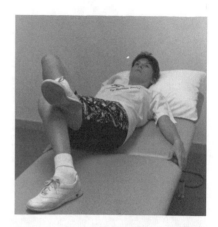

Figure 2.23 Hip abductor stretch.

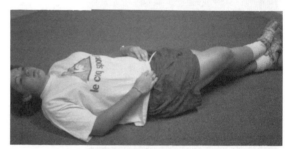

Figure 2.24 Hip abductor
stretch.

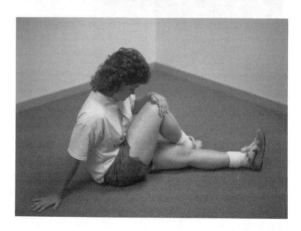

Figure 2.25 Hip abductor
stretch.

unsupported while slightly flexing the knee will emphasize stretching in
the mid-muscle belly, thus removing tension from the popliteal region. The
medial hamstrings are emphasized when the weightbearing extremity is externally rotated (Figure 2.26) and the lateral hamstrings are emphasized when
the weightbearing extremity is internally rotated (Figure 2.27). To stretch the

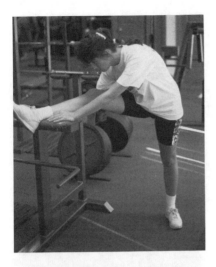

Figure 2.26 Standing medial hamstring stretch.

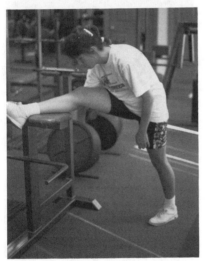

Figure 2.27 Standing lateral hamstring stretch.

distal aspect of the hamstrings, the popliteal area, and the proximal gastrocnemius, the calcaneus should remain supported with the ankle relatively dorsiflexed. This can be performed in multiple positions but is easiest to regulate as demonstrated in Figure 2.28. There are many stretching positions for the hamstrings, including using Figures 2.2 and 2.6 which place more emphasis on the hamstrings than the back extensors if the knees are relatively more extended. If the hamstrings are involved more proximally, any stretches emphasizing the hip extensors should be tried, with the knee *not* fully flexed, as in Figure 2.29.

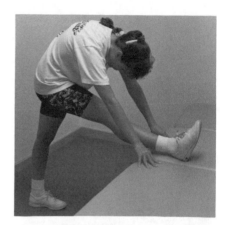

Figure 2.28 Distal hamstring, popliteal and proximal gastrocnemius stretch.

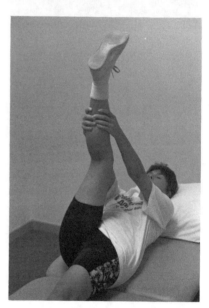

Figure 2.29 Proximal hamstring stretch.

Effectiveness

Stretching is best instructed when the clinician has personal experience with these exercises. I encourage all clinicians to routinely engage in stretching and to experiment with different stretching positions. Unique problems may require modifications for any of these stretches and this can only be achieved through trial and error.

Strengthening

Strength training, as with stretching, depends on sound clinical judgment augmented by personal experience. As with stretching, there is no research that specifically indicates the best exercise program for a given problem. The empirical body of knowledge regarding strength training techniques, however, is substantial. As mentioned previously, bodybuilding and power lifting are two sports where substantial knowledge exists regarding strength training. Weight lifters and weight lifting texts are excellent sources of information for clinicians. The clinician's professional training will augment that information, thus appropriately modifying techniques for specific exercises based on the clinician's judgment regarding the patient.

Training programs for patients differ from training programs for athletes primarily in intensity. All programs must be tailored to the severity of involvement and to the patient's previous experience with exercise. Relatively high repetitions should be used per set when working with patients. This decreases the intensity of the contraction and consequently lowers the risk of reinjury. In the early phases of weight training for patients, the benefit comes not so much from challenging the muscles but rather in training the body to move. In those patients who are extremely deconditioned or fearful, begin with one set of each exercise to minimize normal exercise soreness. In patients who are fearful of what their pain represents or who have limited athletic backgrounds, any experience of discomfort after exercise will be viewed negatively. Consequently, these individuals need to be brought along more slowly. If the patient is in relatively good condition, as judged against a background of LBP patients, begin with two sets per exercise and tell the patient to anticipate some minor exercise-related soreness. Depending on the patient's condition and needs, progress to three sets per exercise after the patient has ceased to experience soreness from two sets and after the weights have been increased so the patient is being relatively more challenged. Typically, my criterion for increasing a patient's weight involves having the patient achieve two or three sets of 15 repetitions per exercise without increased discomfort. Weight is increased in relatively small increments, allowing the patient to achieve at least ten repetitions of the next weight, for two or three sets. The clinician must keep in mind the relative percentage increase in weight. For example, for patients who are lifting 100 pounds, moving them to 110 pounds is only a 10% increase; whereas patients who are lifting 10 pounds change their weight by 100% if they increase the weight to 20 pounds. When patients are using relatively low weights, generally smaller incremental changes should be made. If patients have problems transitioning to the next weight, I sometimes continue with the same weight until they can achieve sets of 20 repetitions, or I prescribe an intermediate weight.

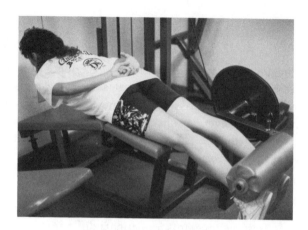

Figure 2.30 Prone supported hyperextension.

Some chronic pain patients will complain of discomfort regardless of the exercise. Further, while many patients with chronic pain report increases in symptoms with increasing activity levels, the study by Linton concludes there is no relationship between activities and reported levels of pain.[33] Therefore, it is important that the clinician and the patient stay very goal oriented. The patient should not achieve 15 repetitions of a given weight and then continue at that weight indefinitely. Some programs fail only because patients are never instructed to advance their weights. At *every* appointment, patients should be encouraged to either increase repetitions or weights.

When beginning the weight training phase of the static exercise program, I typically limit not only the weight, but the number of exercises. This allows accurate identification of problems and facilitates rapid adjustments in the program. Additionally, I may have the patient begin exercises for the purpose of developing mild soreness in uninvolved muscle groups. In patients with chronic LBP, allowing muscles that are not part of the chief complaint to become sore helps patients understand that muscles often become uncomfortable under normal circumstances; therefore, they can anticipate the same will occur with many exercises or activities that involve the back.

In most patients, the four exercises which I initially prescribe include hyperextensions from a slightly flexed prone position, crunches, lateral trunk bends, and dead lifts.

Hyperextension

When performing hyperextensions, the patient begins the exercise with his hands behind his back, extending through pain-free ranges while focusing on the back extensors and not substituting by contracting the hamstrings (Figure 2.30). Once the patient has achieved three sets of 15 repetitions, the same exercise is performed with the hands behind the neck. The

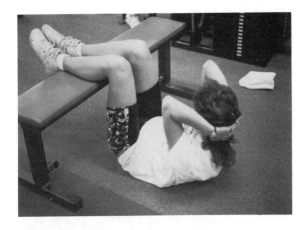

Figure 2.31 Rectus abdominis crunch.

next progression is hyperextensions on a Roman chair, first with hands behind the back and then with hands behind the neck. Resistance can be added by having the patient rest a weight on the interscapular region. If this weight is progressed too aggressively, the patient will substitute by strongly contracting the hamstrings.

Sit-ups

Sit-ups can be performed in multiple positions, all having some benefit. In the early stages, crunches focus on the rectus abdominis while protecting the lumbar spine. This exercise can be performed as noted in Figure 2.31 or several modifications can be used. For each modification, however, the hips are flexed and the lower extremities are not fixed. This minimizes the contribution of the iliopsoas. *Oblique crunches* can be used to improve trunk rotation and strengthen the obliques (Figure 2.32). The exercise should be performed slowly, coming to the end of the range by rotating as much as possible. Patients usually progress in repetitions and intensity of contractions rather than increasing resistance. It is important to remind patients that the cervical spine should not be hyperflexed when performing sit-ups. Full range sit-ups with the lower extremities fixed are more stressful and should not be performed until later stages in the rehabilitation program. While the hip flexors are involved in this exercise, keep in mind that the hip flexors are estimated to produce about 50% of trunk flexion force.[34] Consequently, in fully developing trunk flexion, the contribution of the hip flexors should not be ignored. The most common error made when performing full range sit-ups is keeping the lumbar spine in a neutral or even extended posture while performing the exercise. Performed properly and when patients have developed adequate strength, this exercise does not exacerbate symptoms. There are several good machines on the market that will assist with developing trunk flexion force.

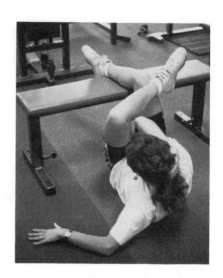

Figure 2.32 Oblique crunch.

Lateral Trunk Bends

When performing lateral trunk bends, I encourage the patient to move through pain-free ranges, initially concentrating on increasing range of motion with a small weight before increasing the resistance (Figure 2.7). The patient needs to be encouraged to maintain strict form without deviating into flexion.

Dead Lifts

Dead lifts are probably the most controversial exercise in the rehabilitation of LBP patients. If properly performed, the motion is safe and is the primary exercise to help prepare for normal lifting activities. Many physicians panic when they hear their patients are performing dead lifts, fearing they will herniate a disc. Patients will certainly reinjure their backs if untrained in this motion.

Initially, dead lifts are performed by using a dumbbell held vertically (Figure 2.8). I transition patients from a 25-pound dumbbell to the 45-pound olympic bar. Though this is a substantial increase in weight, patients are usually lifting well below their capacity when using the 25-pound dumbbell. Even though they notice some increase in weight when lifting the olympic bar, most patients are excited to discover they have just increased their weight by 20 pounds. While this is possible with many patients, again good clinical judgment needs to be used before making such a large increase in weight.

When performing olympic bar dead lifts, the hands should be placed alternately to prevent the bar from rolling. There are two styles of dead lifts: the sumo style, with the legs spread apart and the hands closer together as in

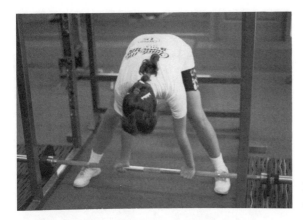

Figure 2.33 Sumo style dead lift.

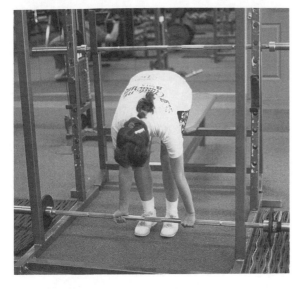

Figure 2.34 Conventional style dead lift.

Figure 2.33, or the conventional style, with the hands spread farther than the lower extremities as depicted in Figure 2.34. Use whichever is most comfortable for the patient.

Other Exercises

While these four exercises make up the core of a patient's program, other exercises must be considered based on the patient's condition. *Seated rows* and *seated pull-downs* are often the next exercises to initiate (Figures 2.35 and 2.36). Usually they are easily tolerated by the patient, placing little stress on the back extensors. A more aggressive exercise that stresses the latissimus dorsi and interscapular muscles while improving

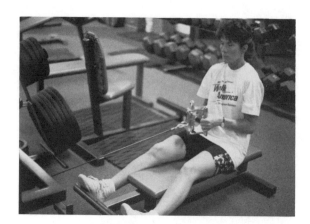

Figure 2.35 Seated rowing.

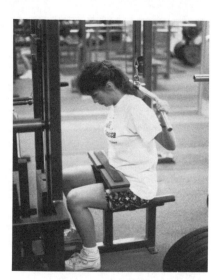

Figure 2.36 Seated pull-downs.

endurance activity in the back extensors is the *bent over row* (Figure 2.37). The advantage of using a machine for bent over rows is the greater range of motion achieved and better control of the weight. Many other variations of this exercise exist.

Another important exercise is the *squat.* Many patients have significant lower extremity weakness, impacting specifically on this motion. As a precursor to full squats, *lateral step-ups* (sometimes called lateral raises) isolate one side and the range of motion can be regulated. A surface any-where from 2 to 8 inches in height can be used, depending on the patient's tolerance. Once the patient progresses to two sets of 20 repetitions off an 8-inch surface, the patient can usually be progressed to full squats. Initially,

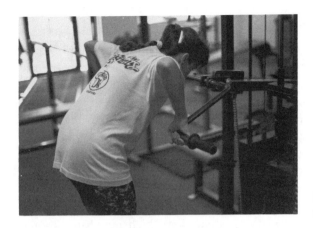

Figure 2.37 Bent over machine row.

squats are performed by holding onto a fixed structure for balance, followed eventually by dumbbell squats (Figure 2.38). I never have patients perform power lifting squats (with an olympic bar resting on the shoulders), as this places a great deal of stress on the back and too many patients will exacerbate their symptoms. Additionally, that particular activity is never routinely encountered.

Other exercises that can be used include straight leg raises, cable hip raises, leg curls, leg extensions, standing calf raises, and many others. Something to be considered, however, is the length of time the patients will be exercising. So as not to increase their workout time unduly, I try not to have them overexercise with peripheral routines that do not directly impact on the trunk.

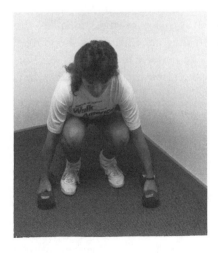

Figure 2.38 Dumbbell squats.

Endurance Training

There are two phases in a patient's endurance training program—the cardiovascular phase and the muscular phase. As indicated in the chapter on muscle fatigue, endurance training is important though *empirically not as well understood* as strength training. Work-hardening programs attempt to address this concern whereas few traditional weight lifting programs target this issue. In helping the patient regain endurance, I typically do not perform endurance muscular training of the back until the patient has already achieved good strength gains. I find clinically that if I begin endurance training the back extensors too early, this seems to inhibit progress with weight training. The exercises that I use for back extensor endurance training include: sustained extension off the Roman chair; high repetition Roman chair hyperextensions; bent over rows; walking; and, in some cases, high repetition dead lifts up to 30 per set for four or five sets. When performing sustained hyperextensions on the Roman chair, the patient monitors the amount of time he is able to maintain that position. I find that there is a good correlation between the patient's ability to tolerate endurance activities at work with the ability to sustain this position. I have rehabilitated patients who could dead lift in excess of 150 pounds and yet were unable to maintain this position for more than 30 seconds. Once they are able to maintain this position for about 80 seconds, their ability to tolerate work-related activities improves substantially. The time for sustained hyperextension can be increased as much as necessary, but typically I try for 2 minutes. Patients perform one set of this exercise at the end of their three-set program of hyperextensions.

I believe walking is an outstanding endurance training activity and I have had patients walk continuously up to four miles as a means of helping them retrain for normal activities. If this seems excessive, consider the amount of time people spend walking when they are Christmas shopping.

Cardiovascular endurance training can be performed on an exercise bicycle, treadmill, stair-training machine, upper extremity ergometer, or whatever other piece of equipment is available in the clinic. I have patients maintain their target heart rate initially in the lower zones, but eventually encourage them to have days when they train in higher zones for the prescribed time frame. I do not usually train people cardiovascularly over 30 minutes but I very rapidly increase their time up to 20 minutes. I find cardiovascular training to be an integral aspect of the patient's back reconditioning program, not because the activity directly influences the back musculature, but because the improved general sense of well-being from the activity seems to carry over. Whether this is attributed to a release of endorphins, improved cardiovascular status, or some other physiologic event, the results clinically are very good and seem to allow patients to improve in all aspects of their program. Heart rate monitoring and, when appropriate, blood pressure monitoring are important aspects in progressing patients. Without heart rate monitors, most patients will underexercise and therefore never achieve the desired benefits.

All exercise prescriptions are best made by individuals who possess personal experience and who consequently can add valuable insight into the patient's experience. Since we do not have adequate research to tell us specifically which programs are most effective, personal experience combined with professional training in anatomy, kinesiology, physiology, and so on provides the ideal marriage of academia with practical knowledge. Clinicians should be aware that lay people are frequently involved in the rehabilitation of patients with LBP. Many health spa employees offer advice on how to recover from a back injury. I have encountered patients who achieved a reasonable degree of success and who, in fact, have stated this has been more helpful than previously prescribed treatment. This is likely due to a premise stated earlier, that exercise, nearly any exercise, is better than none when treating patients with LBP. The prescription of low back pain exercises, however, clearly should be in the hands of skilled clinicians.

Summary

While we may not have adequate research regarding exercise, it is empirically clear that even in the absence of other treatment, exercise can be highly effective. Further, these exercises allow the patient a level of independence in treatment. The clinician does not have to be highly skilled in manual techniques to instruct patients in these exercises and once patients have progressed through the entire program, they have replicated virtually every movement they would likely encounter in any activity.

Exercise prescriptions need to move toward simplicity. Exercises should be easily understood by clinicians and most importantly, by patients. If the program does not make sense empirically, is overly complex based on existing knowledge, or purports miraculous cures, I suggest that clinicians avoid those programs. Claims of remarkable success are unlikely because there are so many uncontrolled variables when dealing with LBP patients. For many of these variables, we have either little control or little knowledge. Most patients' successes will come about as a result of a well-thought-out clinical program of treatment combined with a high degree of motivation and confidence on the part of the patient. The programs described in this chapter are simple and combine current research with empirical knowledge. This is not to say that these exercises are the only way to treat patients with LBP; however, they provide a place to begin.

References

1. Haldeman S: Presidential Address, North American Spine Society: Failure of the pathology model to predict back pain. Spine 15:7 718–724, 1990.
2. Saal JA, Saal JS: Rehabilitation of the patient, in White AH and Anderson R, (eds) Conservative Care of Low Back Pain. Baltimore, Williams and Wilkins, 21–29, 1991.
3. Spitzer WO, LeBlanc FE, Dupuis M: Scientific approach to the assessment and management of activity-related spinal disorders. Spine 12:7 1–59, 1987.
4. Williams PC: Lesions of the lumbosacral spine, Part I. J Bone Joint Surg 19:343–363, 1937.
5. Williams PC: Lesions of the lumbosacral spine, Part II. J Bone Joint Surg 19:690–703, 1937.
6. Ponte DJ, Jensen MA, Kent BE: A preliminary report on the use of the McKenzie protocol versus Williams protocol in the treatment of low back pain. J Orthop Sports Phys Ther 6:130–139, 1984.
7. Flint MM: Effect of increasing back and abdominal muscle strength on low back pain. Res Quart 24:2 160–171, 1955.
8. Davies JE, Gibson T, Tester L: The value of exercises in the treatment of low back pain. Rheumatol Rehabil 19:243–247, 1979.
9. Kendall PH, Jenkins JM: Exercises for backache: A double-blind controlled trial. Physiotherapy 54:154–157, 1968.
10. Mitchell RI, Carmen GM: Results of a multi-centered trial using an intensive active exercise program for the treatment of acute soft tissue and back injuries. Spine 15:6 514–521, 1990.
11. Fordyce WE, McMahon R, Rainwater G, et al: Pain complaint: Exercise performance relationship in chronic pain. Pain 10:311–321, 1981.
12. Mayer TG, Gatchel RJ, Kishino N, et al: Objective assessment of spine function following industrial injury: A prospective study with comparison group and one-year follow-up. Spine 10:482–493, 1985.
13. Alston W, Carlson KE, Feldman D, et al: A quantitative study of muscle factors in the chronic low-back syndrome. J Am Ger Soc 14:10 1041–1047, 1966.
14. Nachemson A, Lindh M: Measurement of abdominal and back muscle strength with and without low back pain. Scand J Rehab Med 1:60–69, 1969.
15. Thorstensson A, Arvidson A: Trunk muscle strength and low back pain. Scand J Rehab Med 14:69–75, 1982.
16. McNeill T, Warwick D, Andersson G, Ashultz A: Trunk strengths in attempted flexion, extension and lateral bending in healthy subjects and patients with low-back disorders. Spine 5:6 529–538, 1980.

17. Kishino ND, Mayer TG, Gatchel RJ, et al: Quantification of lumbar function, Part IV: Isometric and isokinetic lifting simulation in normal subjects and low-back dysfunction patients. Spine 10:10 921–927, 1985.
18. Cady L, Bischoff D, O'Connel E, et al: Strength and fitness and subsequent back injuries in firefighters. J Occup Med 21(4):269–279, 1979.
19. Nicolaisen T, Jorgensen T: Trunk strength, back muscle endurance and low-back trouble. Scan J Rehab Med 14:121–127, 1985.
20. Jorgensen K, Nicolaisen T: Trunk extensor endurance: Determination and relation to low-back trouble. Ergonomics 30:2 259–267, 1987.
21. Chaffin, DB: Human strength capability and low back pain. J Occup Med 16:248–254, 1974.
22. Keyserling WM, Herrin GD, Chaffin DB: Isometric strength testing as a means of controlling medical incidents on strenuous jobs. J Occup Med 22:332–336, 1980.
23. Troup JDG, Martin JW, Lloyd DCEF: Back pain in industry: A prospective survey. Spine 6:61–69, 1981.
24. Nachemson A, Lindh M: Measurement of abdominal and back muscle strength with and without low back pain. Scand J Rehab Med 1:60–65, 1969.
25. Leino P, Aro S, Hasan J: Trunk muscle function and low-back disorders: A 10-year follow-up study. J Chron Dis 40:4 289–296, 1987.
26. Gonnella C, Paris SP, Kutner M: Reliability in Evaluating Passive Intervertebral Motion. Phys Ther 62:436–444, 1982.
27. Kaltenborn F, Lindahl O: Reproducerbarheten Vid Rorelsundersckning Av Enskilda Kotor. Lakartidningen 6:962–965, 1969.
28. McNab I: The traction spur: An indicator of segmental instability. J Bone Joint Surg 53–A:4 663–670, 1971.
29. Gertzbein SD, Seligman J, Holtby R, et al: Centrode patterns and segmental instability in degenerative disc disease. Spine 10:3 257–261, 1985.
30. Silberstein CE: The evolution of degenerative changes in the cervical spine and an investigation into the "joints of luschka." Clin Orthop 40:184–204, 1965.
31. Witt, I, Vestergaard A, Rosenklint A: A comparative analysis of X-ray findings of the lumbar spine in patients with and without lumbar pain. Spine 19:3 298–300, 1984.
32. Walker ML, Rothstein JM, Finucane SD, Lamb RL: Relationships between lumbar lordosis, pelvic tilt and abdominal muscle performance. Phys Ther 67:4 512–516, 1987.
33. Linton SJ: The relationship between activity and chronic back pain. Pain 21:289–294, 1985.
34. Langrana NA, Lee CK: Isokinetic evaluation of trunk muscles. Spine 9:2 287–290, 1984.

3

□ □ □
□ □ □
□ □ □

Rehabilitation after Back Surgery

Ronald C. Childs
Gunnar B. J. Andersson

All patients are not the same and surgical procedures vary. For those reasons, postoperative rehabilitation is not uniform, but varies from case to case. Certain principles apply to all situations, however. Those principles will be stressed in this chapter, but by no means represent the only approach. There is little science in this area. Basic knowledge about the healing of tissue, common sense, and empirical results provide the basis of postoperative rehabilitation. The principles discussed in this chapter have proven to be rewarding, safe, and acceptable to the patient, as well as easy to implement.

Postoperative rehabilitation begins preoperatively whenever possible. A well-conditioned patient with only minor loss of physical function will recover faster from the surgical trauma and thus will present less of a problem when attempting to restore full function postoperatively. The patient's psychological state and motivation are also critical and can be influenced preoperatively. Preparing the patient for the sometimes long and demanding postoperative rehabilitation is as important as explaining the nature of the surgical procedure. Frequently, the patient believes the problem will be solved by the procedure alone only to find that the operation, in fact, is only the beginning of the end.

In spinal surgery, as in other surgical procedures, the speed with which rehabilitation can be implemented depends on the need to protect different tissues during the healing process and the wish to start using the tissues functionally as early as possible. Again, there is little information about when precisely the optimal endpoint of healing and the starting point of functional use begins. In general, healing time (defined in those terms) occurs earlier than was previously believed. Therefore, activity should resume earlier than was often the case in the past. Also, nonoperated organs such as the heart, lungs, and peripheral vascular system and other body parts (legs and arms) can be stressed beneficially from the beginning without interfering with the healing process of the spinal tissues. The nature of the surgical procedure is critical in the decision-making process. Clearly a different approach is needed for a patient who has undergone a microdiscectomy and one who has had a fusion.

This chapter provides the framework and principles for rehabilitation after back surgery onto which individual approaches can be grafted. As such, we limit the discussion to the lumbar spine and concentrate our efforts on the discussion of rehabilitation after disc hernia procedures, laminectomies and fusions for spinal stenosis, and spondylolisthesis.

General Principles

Postoperative rehabilitation falls into three phases: early postoperative care, physical rehabilitation, and vocational rehabilitation. There are no strict borders between these phases. Rather, they are most efficiently integrated and interfaced with each other. Vocational issues should be discussed with the patient preoperatively to ensure realistic expectations. Most patients can return to their regular job after simple disc procedures, while for some patients requiring other procedures this would be ill advised, even with good surgical results.

Pain management is crucial to effective rehabilitation. In the early postoperative period narcotics are almost always indicated, but for a short period only. These drugs are administered by intermittent intramuscular injections, continuous infusion, or by patient-controlled analgesia pumps. This latter technique has become popular since it provides medication when needed and requires a smaller overall dose than intermittent or continuous infusions. Narcotics should be discontinued rapidly and replaced by oral analgesics and/ or nonsteroidal anti-inflammatory drugs. In patients with fusions, NSAIDs should be avoided because they interfere with the bone healing process.

Once antibiotic prophylaxis and intravenous medication needs are met, intravenous access may be discontinued. A urinary bladder catheter, if present, should be removed as soon as possible. Bed rest, narcotics, and pain may make straight catheterization necessary. Wound drains are typically removed in 24 to 48 hours. Following anterior fusion, nasogastric suction is usually necessary but is removed as bowel activity returns.

Irrespective of procedure, mobilization after surgery should be rapid. This reduces the risk of complications from the lungs and from the peripheral vascular system such as emboli and deep vein thromboses. Breathing exercises should be started immediately, and patients should be encouraged to "pump" with their feet. We routinely begin beside "dangling" on the first postoperative day and standing and walking on the first or second postsurgical day. Patients then progress rapidly to a level of activity that allows them to return home. Most patients reach this level easily in two to five days depending on the procedure. They need help initially, which can often be provided by a floor nurse. The guidance of a physical therapist is always helpful, but is not an absolute requirement. Discharge instructions should be clear and detailed with respect to activities; written instructions are always helpful. If the patients have not had preoperative instructions, then simple maneuvers such as getting in and out of bed and chairs must be taught during the hospital period.

Preoperative Management

The importance of the preoperative management cannot be overstated due to its significant impact on the postoperative course. Patients should be educated regarding their condition and the indications for and nature of the planned procedure should be explained in detail. It is imperative that the need for active participation by the patient in his or her care is fully explained and that realistic goals are set.

Nutritional status is frequently overlooked, yet its effect on the outcome of surgery is well documented. Poor nutritional status is associated with increased mortality and complications such as infection, wound dehiscence, and delay in mobilization. Bone healing is greatly influenced by nutritional status. The need for a specific nutritional evaluation in elective surgery is uncommon, but is indicated by a serum albumin level of 3.4 mg/dl or less, a total lymphocyte count of less than 1500, anergy to skin testing, or unexplained recent weight loss. Body weight alone is not an adequate indicator of nutritional status.

Elderly patients often have other medical problems and should be medically evaluated and cleared prior to elective surgery. Smokers should be educated regarding the detrimental effects of tobacco usage. This is particularly important in cases where a fusion is planned. Bone healing is negatively influenced by smoking, and increased rates of pseudoarthroses are associated with this habit. Patients are also instructed to stop taking NSAIDs prior to surgery to avoid coagulation problems. Because the half-life of NSAIDs vary greatly, the interval period between when to stop and the time of the procedure may vary. Typically, at least 48 hours is recommended.

Tissue Healing

Tissue healing is a dynamic process that begins at wound closure and continues well after the incision is healed. Soft tissue healing may be divided into three phases which represent a continuum of events—the inflammatory phase, the collagen (repair) phase, and the maturation (remodeling) phase.

The inflammatory phase is the initial response of the body to the trauma of surgery and usually lasts three to four days. The area of the incision is characterized by cut tissues, blood vessels, and so on, with the resultant formation of cellular debris. Vasoactive substances (histamine, serotonin) are immediately released and cause increased vascular dilatation and permeability, allowing polymorphonuclear leucocytes to enter the involved area. As the process continues, additional mediators of inflammation including prostaglandins are released and the leucocyte population becomes predominantly lymphocytes, macrophages, and monocytes. These cells function to remove the necrotic by-products created by the surgical trauma.

The collagen or repair phase is characterized by vascular capillary ingrowth into the wound and a rapid increase in fibroblastic collagen production. This process peaks by seven to ten days postoperatively and slows by the end of the second week. Although there is abundant collagen in the wound, maximal tensile strength has not been attained because the collagen is poorly organized, poorly oriented (not along lines of stress), and immature with minimal cross-linking between fibers. However, due to the abundance of collagen, skin suture or staples may be removed at this time. In many patients, resorbable intracutaneous sutures are used to close the skin. These, of course, should be left alone until they resorb, which takes many weeks.

During the maturation phase, collagen remodeling is occurring. The fibers become organized and oriented along lines of tension and cross-linking is accomplished (Figure 3.1).[1] This eventually results in maximum tensile strength of the wound. This process begins at around fourteen days and may last several months. The process is positively influenced by controlled activity.

Muscular repair occurs by a similar process. The initial cellular inflammatory response is followed by scar tissue formation in the first postoperative week. Animal studies indicate that muscles can already produce active tension at this time. If the surgical incision goes across muscle fibers, muscle must regenerate across the repair site for normal function to occur. This is rarely completely successful and is why, in spinal procedures, muscle is preferably stripped off from the bony insertion rather than cut directly. The innervation of muscle tissue is also less damaged by this technique, although electromyographic (EMG) studies of back muscles after surgery typically show denervation potentials for a long time. Accumulated experimental evidence shows that protective motion aids in the repair process of muscle as in other tissue.

Discs heal slowly because of their cartilaginous nature and lack of vascular supply. Fibroblasts and collagen provide the initial repair, with gradual metaplasia to cartilage occurring over months to years. Vascular ingrowth

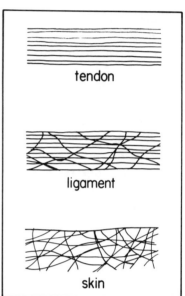

Figure 3.1 During the healing phase, collagen tissue organizes along the lines of tension. The organizational structure of skin is more random than that of fascia, ligament, and tendon. (Adapted from Frankel VF, Nordin M: Basic Biomechanics of the Skeletal System. Philadelphia, Lea and Febiger, 1980.)

occurs in the disc defect and the tissue does not remodel into its original structure. Passive motion has been found to facilitate cartilage repair in articular cartilage, but no such information is available for disc tissue.

Bone healing is similar in many respects to soft tissue healing and there are again three phases. Bone healing is relevant only when a fusion is performed. The objective of a fusion is to create a bony bridge from one spinal motion segment to one or more additional segments so as to restrict motion and impart stability. In preparation for the fusion, a raw bleeding bony surface is created to host the transplanted bone by decorticating elements already present; then bone graft is added. The initial response in bone healing is again to remove the localized tissue debris, which takes much longer in bone than in soft tissue. This resorption occurs by vascular invasion. The bone graft provides a stimulus for bone formation and serves as a lattice for the replacement by living bone. This occurs through a process called creeping substitution, in which new bone forms along the new vascular channels.

Tissue production occurs in the collagen phase, progressing from fibrous to cartilaginous to bone. Newly formed bone has a disorganized structure and is not as strong as the finally remodeled lamellar bone. During the remodeling phase, immature bone is gradually replaced by organized lamellar bone and the definitive fusion is achieved. This process is usually well advanced by four to six months, but may take a year or longer to complete. The graft functions long before this process is completed, however. Surgeons who prescribe braces following lumbar fusions typically prescribe their use for 4

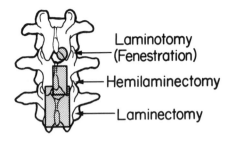
Laminotomy (Fenestration)
Hemilaminectomy
Laminectomy

Figure 3.2 Amount of bone removed in different surgical procedures. (Adapted from Andersson GBJ, McNeill TW: Lumbar Spinal Syndromes. Wien, Springer-Verlag, 1989.)

to 6 months, by which time the fusion mass is believed to be mature enough to no longer require protection. Bone healing is stimulated by mechanical factors, but too much movement can result in a breakup of the fusion mass and pseudarthrosis (incomplete healing). This is the main reason for bracing and also for the use of internal fixation in some procedures. Bone healing is negatively affected by smoking, indicating that smoking cessation is beneficial when a fusion is contemplated.

Postoperative Management

Disc Hernia Procedures

A variety of procedures exist to remove the herniated lumbar disc once a decision to actively intervene is made. These include true laminectomy, limited approach discectomy, microdiscectomy, percutaneous discectomy, chymopapain injections, and laser discectomy (Figure 3.2).[2] A true laminectomy is performed for disc hernias only when a cauda equina syndrome is present or the disc hernia is so large that more access is required. The rehabilitation for these few patients is as described under stenosis, or if the laminectomy is small, as with laminotomy. Laminectomy and discectomy usually involve a mid-line incision 3 to 6 cm. in length at the level of the involved disc space. The paraspinal musculature is elevated subperiosteally from the spinous processes and laminae on the involved side and the ligamentum flavum is dissected and removed to expose the dura and the nerve root. The root is mobilized and usually retracted medially and the disc is entered at the site of herniation. Sometimes a disc fragment has extruded from the disc and an opening is present. In other cases, the herniation is contained by the longitudinal ligament and annular fibers and an incision is necessary before disc tissue can be removed.

Microdiscectomy involves a smaller incision than the standard discectomy and the use of a microscope. The use of headlights and magnifying loupes makes the limited approach discectomy very similar to the microdiscectomy. Thus, these terms are sometimes used synonymously. With percutaneous discectomy, a guide needle is inserted into the involved disc space well lateral to the midline and under radiographic (fluoroscopic) visualization. An aspiration/cutting cannula is inserted over the guide and following radiographic confirmation, the discectomy is performed. A rotating cutting blade "chops" the disc material into small pieces which are aspirated by a mechanical suction device. A laser can be used instead and the disc material removed by this method; this technique is called laser discectomy. Most patients undergo percutaneous discectomy or laser discectomy on an outpatient basis. Chemonucleolysis involves placing a needle in the disc space via the lateral approach and injecting chymopapain. Chymopapain is a proteolytic enzyme that dissolves the disc. The patient is typically discharged the day after the injection.

Disc surgery influences the stability of the motion segment. Research on in vitro specimens has consistently shown decreased stability in lumbar discs following discectomy. The instability increases with the amount of disc material removed and is greatest following total discectomy. Therefore, most surgeons, while taking care to remove all free fragments, excise as little of the annular disc material as possible. The least stable motions in the laboratory were found to be lateral bending and axial rotation. These motions, therefore, should be minimized postoperatively. Extension is the most stable position of an operated disc, making it more reasonable to prescribe extension exercises. There is no universal agreement on how much a patient's musculature can correct or compensate for the postdiscectomy instability.

The alternatives to the standard open discectomy have all been designed to decrease the amount of tissue dissection required, minimize the amount of disc material removed, decrease postoperative pain, decrease hospital stays, and increase the rate at which patients can be mobilized following the surgical trauma.

Animal studies have been used to study the effects of chemonucleolysis. Increased disc flexibility/instability has been noted up to 2 weeks following injection in animals with the largest increase noted in flexion. By 6 months, lateral flexion motion has returned to normal, but flexion and torsion flexibility remain increased.

Following a standard limited approach discectomy, patients are allowed out of bed the first postoperative day and, if comfortable, may ambulate wearing a canvas corset. Diet is advanced as tolerated and IV fluids are discontinued as rapidly as possible. Prophylactic antibiotics are continued for 12 hours postoperatively. During hospitalization, therapy is initiated to improve gait, mobility, and endurance. Early mobility is actually associated with decreased use of pain medications, probably through activation of the patient's endogenous endorphin system. The patient is typically discharged on the third postoperative day with a limited amount of narcotics prescribed for pain.

Conditioning is emphasized in the first postoperative period at home. Walking is encouraged as it is easy to implement and nonstressful to the spine. We recommend walking at least one mile per day. Long-term sitting (at home and in cars), bending, twisting, and lifting are discouraged. Sports are not recommended for 6 weeks but isometric exercises of the abdominals, gluteals, and thigh musculature are encouraged. Swimming can start after the wound has healed. It is usually easier to swim using back strokes than other swim techniques. Stationary bikes are also excellent tools at this stage.

Return to work depends on the type of work performed. Patients with sedentary jobs may return to work, at least part-time, 2 to 3 weeks postoperatively. Heavy laborers may require 6 to 12 weeks before resuming work. All patients should have formal physical therapy to strengthen the trunk and leg muscles, reinforce the importance of good body mechanics, and learn a home exercise program to be continued for life. Heavy laborers may benefit from a subsequent work hardening program. This is particularly true if there has been a significant time period out of work. These patients are frequently severely deconditioned.

Chymopapain patients are typically discharged the following day with a lumbosacral corset. The rehabilitation is similar to that of a patient after a limited approach discectomy. Percutaneous lumbar discectomy patients who obtain immediate relief from sciatic pain may return to sedentary jobs 1 to 2 weeks postoperatively. Patients are usually discharged the day of surgery with pain medication prescribed. Rehabilitation is again similar to that with a standard discectomy.

Spinal Stenosis

Patients with lumbar spinal stenosis are frequently elderly and, as previously mentioned, should receive a complete and thorough medical evaluation preoperatively. Patients typically undergo a wide, frequently multiple-level decompressive laminectomy.[3] Fusion is performed when instability is present or is created by the decompression.

In cases where decompression only is performed, the patient is allowed to dangle at bedside postoperatively on day one and walk to the bathroom under supervision. Additional ambulation, at first with assistance, is encouraged by the second postoperative day and the patient is fitted with a lumbosacral corset. If a fusion is performed, the process is the same; however, in our institution, the patient wears a low profile thoraco-lumbar-spinal orthosis (regardless of whether instrumentation is used). Some surgeons do not routinely brace their patients postoperatively, whether or not fusion is performed. We do, believing that initially there is less pain and, in the case of fusion, there is a need for stabilization during the healing period. Mobilization increases rapidly during the hospital stay and patients are typically discharged 5 to 7 days after surgery. We do not use physical therapy routinely, although this would be an advantage. By the time patients are discharged, they are comfortable, walking a reasonable distance and up and down stairs, as well as completing basic activities of daily living. Discharge planning should include visiting nurses and homemaker aides as needed. Outpatient physical therapy is rarely needed initially because the main emphasis is on conditioning and endurance. Walking is encouraged with specific goals set for the patient. Because walking may be uncomfortable at first, the exercise bike provides an attractive alternative. This is particularly true in climates where cold, snow, rain, or extreme heat sometimes make outdoor walking a problem. Aquatic exercises or simply walking in water are also excellent alternatives when wound healing is complete.

We do not emphasize muscle strengthening exercises during the first 2 to 3 months after wide laminectomies, and not until healing is complete in spinal fusions. This does not mean that upper or lower extremity exercises are not permitted, simply that they are not emphasized. Most of our patients are elderly and need to concentrate on conditioning rather than on muscle strengthening or flexibility.

As patients' endurance and mobility increases, the focus should switch to increasing strength (via physical therapy, walking, and swimming). This will typically begin at about 4 to 6 weeks postoperatively. Patients who have sedentary jobs may be able to return to work at least on a part-time basis at this time. Those with physically demanding jobs should have continued emphasis on reconditioning through walking, biking, swimming, and so on. By 6 months, patients who are heavy laborers should be enrolled in an active physical therapy program followed by a work hardening program and subsequent return to their previous occupation when possible. Initially, work return may be light duty, possibly part-time with full unlimited duty resumed gradually. If this is not feasible and patients cannot return to their previous occupation, a work capacity evaluation (functional evaluation) should be performed to determine what type of work patients can perform. This provides a basis for modified work return or vocational efforts.

Orthotics

Orthotics are not necessary in all patients operated on for spinal conditions. Special precautions are necessary, however, in patients who have had wide multilevel decompressions in order to reduce the risk of late fracture of the pars interarticularis or remaining facet. We fit these patients with a custom-made thoraco-lumbar orthosis (Figure 3.3). In patients who have not had a fusion but may be at risk of fracture, use of the orthosis is continued for 6 to 12 weeks. For patients who have had a fusion, the brace

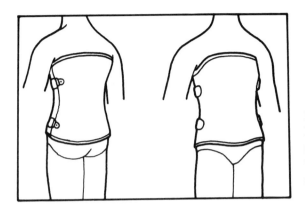

Figure 3.3 Thoraco-lumbar orthosis. (Adapted from Andersson GBJ, McNeill TW: Lumbar Spinal Stenosis. St. Louis, Mosby Year Book, 1992.)

treatment is continued until the fusion shows good consolidation by X-ray. For patients who have undergone spinal instrumentation (internal fixation), we still feel that the use of a postoperative orthosis is important, particularly when the bone is osteoporotic. The risk of bony failure at the attachment sites for the instrumentation (screws, hooks, and so on) increases rapidly as the bone becomes more osteoporotic. Further, the risk of failure above the instrumented level is also great due to increased stress concentration on the segment adjacent to the rigidly instrumented level. Bracing is intended to reduce the risk of screw or hook detachment and to lower the stress concentration at the unfused segments while allowing physical rehabilitation to progress otherwise.

The need for orthotics after spinal operations is controversial and there are no clean prospective scientific studies. A lumbar orthosis cannot prevent intervertebral motions and can only mildly reduce the load on the spine. However, by keeping the trunk upright, gross motions and the overall load can be kept at a minimum. Micromotion is probably an important factor with respect to the healing of a fusion. Recent studies by Johnsson et al.[4] using internal markers and Roentgen stereophotogrammatic analysis (RSA) revealed that translations between fused vertebrae begin to decrease 3 to 6 months after a successful noninstrumented posterolateral fusion (Figures 3.4 and 3.5). By 12 months, the fusion was considered rigid. The use of rigid orthoses for 5 months resulted in a significantly higher fusion rate than when the same orthosis was used for only 3 months. Apparently the consolidation of a fusion takes as long as 6 months. Based on this information, we prefer to keep our fused patients in a brace for 6 months postoperatively.

Electric stimulation is increasingly used to promote healing of spinal fusions. Direct current stimulation has been demonstrated to enhance fusion in nonblinded and nonrandomized clinical studies,[5] and a randomized double-blind prospective study of pulsed electromagnetic fields for lumbar

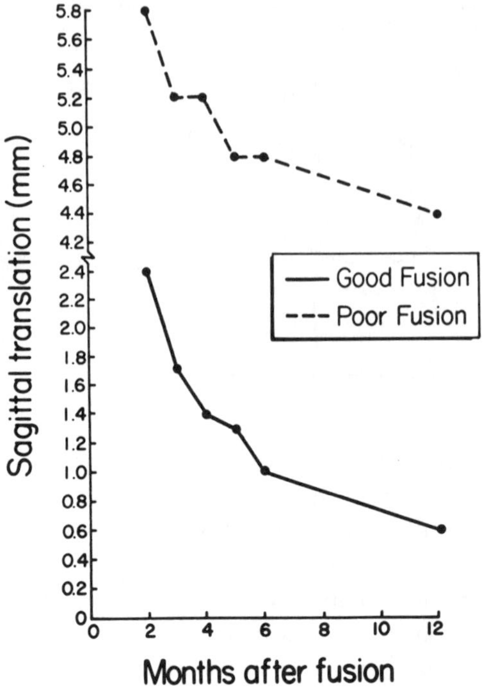

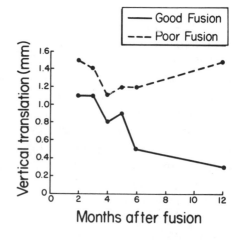

Figure 3.4 Mean sagittal translation on flexion-extension views between vertebrae determined by Roentgen stereophotogrammetry. Ten fusions with good results compared to ten with poor fusion. (Adapted from Johnsson R, Stromquist B, Axelsson P, et al: Influence of spinal immobilization on consolidation of posterolateral fusion. Spine 17:16–21, 1992.)

anterior interbody fusions showed significantly higher fusion rates for active versus inactive treatment (92% success versus 65%).[6] We have used pulsed electromagnetic stimulation over the past 7 years, with excellent results and compliance for all types of fusions, but have not performed a randomized evaluation of its use.

Figure 3.5 Mean vertical translation between the ten good and poor fusions studied with Roentgen stereophotogrammetry. (Adapted from Johnsson R, Stromquist B, Axelsson P, et al: Influence of spinal immobilization on consolidation of posterolateral fusion. Spine 17:16–21, 1992.

Vocational Issues

Patients with chronic pain are frequently depressed and may benefit from psychological or psychiatric intervention preoperatively and postoperatively. While it is important to provide appropriate analgesia in the initial postoperative period, patients should be weaned from narcotics as rapidly as possible. The time will vary with the patient and the procedure performed. Physical rehabilitation will frequently be uncomfortable and patient education with realistic goal selection is essential to allow patients to actively participate in their own care.

The vocational goal is to return the worker to the workplace and, ideally, to his or her previous occupation. This may require worksite modification or permanent activity limitations. If this is not feasible, a new position must be sought and additional training provided. For the elderly stenotic patient, the goal may be to resume a more active and rewarding lifestyle free of the experienced pain restrictions and decreased ambulatory status.

Summary

The care of the spine surgery patient is a multidisciplinary effort requiring input from the patient, the surgeon, nurses, physical therapists, vocational/rehabilitation specialists, and others. The process starts well before surgery and continues after all procedures are performed. A host of issues—medical, vocational, and so on—must be addressed to provide the best possible chance for functional restoration of the patient.

References

1. Frankel VF, Nordin M: Basic Biomechanics of the Skeletal System. Philadelphia, Lea and Febiger, 1980.
2. Andersson GBJ, McNeill TW: Lumbar Spinal Syndromes. Wien, Springer-Verlag, 1989.
3. Andersson GBJ, McNeill TW: Lumbar Spinal Stenosis. St. Louis, Mosby-Year Book, 1992.
4. Johnsson R, Stromquist B, Axelsson P et al: Influence of spinal immobilization on consolidation of posterolateral fusion. Spine 17:16–21, 1992.
5. Kane WT: Direct current electrical bone stimulation for spinal fusion. Spine B:763–765, 1988.
6. Mooney V: A randomized double-blind prospective study of the efficacy of pulsed electromagnetic fields for interbody lumbar fusions. Spine 15:708–712, 1990.

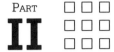

Assessment and Management Strategies

The study of psychosocial dysfunction has offered many answers to clinicians frustrated by varying patient responses to identical treatment techniques for similar physiologic dysfunctions. In the past, much of the variation in response had wrongly been attributed to overly simplistic classifications such as "compensationitis." Other similarly punitive labels failed to recognize the complex psychosocial dynamics involved in the pain experience. The need for psychological support personnel has become increasingly evident with research confirming that specific psychosocial variables are better prognostic indicators for low back pain treatment outcomes than many physiologic signs.

Chapter 4, Psychological Assessment Strategies for Low Back Pain Patients in the Physical Therapy Setting examines how a clinician can recognize barriers to successful rehabilitation and avoid the pitfalls of overly simplistic labeling. As the pain experience is explored, cognitive and behavioral issues are presented to help delineate the responsibilities of both clinicians and patients in the recovery process.

Many clinical mistakes can perpetuate the patient's chronic pain complaint. Psychosocial assessment provides a base for the development of specific management strategies to avoid these mistakes and improve rehabilitation outcomes. Chapter 5, Chronic Pain: Treatment Considerations, presents successful experiences using motivational techniques, dialogues to use and avoid, and utilization of functional measures to guide the patient's successful rehabilitation are presented with numerous clinical examples. Equally important, the reader will learn to recognize that psychosocial dysfunctions may be interfering with a clinician's best efforts to help the patient. This chapter will provide clinicians with information regarding why they should refer a patient to a mental health professional as well as when and to whom the patient should be referred.

A specific outgrowth of psychosocial assessment and research is the often misunderstood term "symptom magnification syndrome." Chapter 6, "Managing Symptom Magnification," takes a functionally oriented approach to symptom magnification while providing specific dialogue to use with patients to keep their rehabilitation moving in a positive direction. In combining the specific information on symptom magnification syndrome with psychological assessment and management strategies, this text provides the clinician with an integrated whole which recognizes that successful patient outcomes are often attributable more to sound management strategies than specific physical interventions.

4 ⬜⬜⬜ ⬜⬜⬜ ⬜⬜⬜

Psychological Assessment Strategies for Low Back Pain Patients in the Physical Therapy Setting

Timothy C. Toomey

What Is Pain?

One of the difficulties facing anyone who writes on the topic of pain is how to define it. Perhaps one of the obstacles to formulating a satisfactory definition of pain is its dual nature as a sensory phenomenon common to all organisms endowed with a central nervous system and as an experiential phenomenon that is intensely private and unique and that renders suffering its highly personalized character.[1] Reference to the dictionary seems to support this dualistic view of pain, stating that the term *pain* shares word roots with terms such as cold, choking, and gnawing but also with terms such as punishment, suffering, and being defeated in battle.[2] Thus, it appears that any adequate understanding of pain requires an appreciation of its physiologic and affective/reactive components.

The clinical assessment and treatment of patients with pain, especially chronic pain, is likewise complicated by definitional issues. In medical parlance this is termed the *pain taxonomy problem*. This is related to discipline-specific etiologic theories of pain and often conflicting recommendations and poor communications among the specialists called to consult on the case. A pain clinician recently compared the current understanding of the patient with chronic pain to the classical fable of the blind men and the elephant. That is, each expert called to evaluate the patient is convinced of the accuracy and sufficiency of his or her unique perspective, resulting in a distorted view of the problem and fragmented patterns of patient care. Thus, even among the pain "experts" there is a tendency to confound the sensory and experiential dimensions of pain to the detriment of both patient management and growth of theory and research.

This chapter explores the role and utility of psychological assessment strategies for pain in the clinical setting. It does not encourage clinicians to assume the role of psychologists or to alter in any fundamental manner their traditional skills of patient assessment. It provides the clinician with a multidisciplinary perspective on the problem of pain assessment, an invitation to include a wider range of data in the evaluation of the patient, and encouragement to develop consultative relationships between health care practitioners and psychologists on individual patients with chronic pain.

Developments in Theory and Clinical Practice Relating to Pain Assessment

An early theoretical model of pain was developed by Descartes[3] and termed *specificity theory.* It defined pain in rather simplistic and closed fashion as a registration in consciousness of a noxious sensation that is directly proportional and specific to the amount of peripheral noxious stimulation—that is, nociception. A major shift in the understanding of pain occurred in the mid 1960s with the proposal of the gate control theory of pain by Melzack and Wall.[4] This theory, which attempted to bridge the sensory and experiential dimensions of pain, hypothesized a modulation or "gating" of peripheral nociceptive input in the dorsal horn cells of the spinal cord. Additionally, it proposed that cortical factors could influence the operation of the spinal gate via a "central control trigger." Although subsequent research, including the identification of peripheral sensory[5] and humoral[6] nociceptive systems, has challenged some of the specific postulates of the theory, it continues to be viable in a modified form [7,8] and it has had a profound influence on the understanding of pain in the scientific and medical communities. One result is the importance of evaluating the impact of individual differences, including emotional status, cognitive appraisal, environment, and learning history, on the perception of and response to pain.

Parallel to the theoretical developments in the understanding of pain mechanisms, a practical, clinical approach to evaluating and treating patients with *chronic pain* was being developed by Dr. John Bonica and colleagues at the University of Washington Medical Center. This *multidisci-*

plinary pain clinic concept entailed evaluations of the patient with chronic pain by a number of interested specialists including an anesthesiologist, psychologist/psychiatrist, physical therapist, occupational therapist, and vocational rehabilitation counselor. Then, most importantly, the varying assessments of the patient were shared in a staff meeting attended by all the specialists and an individual treatment plan was developed. The role of behavioral factors was considered to be crucial in this multidisciplinary approach and existing behavioral assessment and treatment methods traditionally employed in the psychiatric setting were modified for use with chronic pain and illness.[9]

Expanding the Dimensions of Pain

One of the results of the theoretical and clinical developments of the 1960s was an expansion in the number of conceptual models for understanding pain. These new models in turn affected strategies of assessment and treatment. We will focus on conceptual expansions of two dimensions of pain given developmental impetus by the gate control theory, stages of pain and models of pain, and examine their impact on our current approaches to evaluate strategies for low back pain rehabilitation.

Stages of Pain: Assessment Implications

The traditional view of pain as a sensory signal reflective of tissue damage which is registered in consciousness and followed by an antinociceptive motor response is an accurate view of pain as an adaptive, biological survival system. Clearly the chest pain that heralds an impending heart attack or the sharp, stabbing pains in the side associated with a perforated appendix represent powerful biological signals of acute tissue damage requiring immediate response. However, the simplistic application of this model to all types of pain results in inappropriate methods of evaluation and treatment.

One of the reasons Melzack cited for his interest in developing a new model for pain was the existence of certain pain conditions where there was an obvious lack of correlation between degree of tissue injury and report of pain, namely, congenital insensitivity to pain, phantom pain, and spontaneous pain. It is the latter group, those with spontaneous pain in the absence of obvious nociceptive input, who frequently progress to a life of chronic suffering, often compounded by environmental factors including the health care system itself. The importance of understanding pain as a progressively developing disorder is reflected in the provision of a separate axis for the evaluation of temporal patterning of pain in the recently proposed pain taxonomy published by the International Association for the Study of Pain.[10] The boundary of this temporal division between acute and chronic pain has traditionally been set at 6 months. However, this is clearly an arbitrary division and the relevant distinction is between pain that is a sensory signal reflective of tissue injury and pain that engenders a series of dysfunctional behavioral and emotional responses.

Development of Chronic Pain: Differing Views

The processes underlying the progression in the stages of pain have been explained in several ways. Hendler emphasizes the establishment of abnormal psychological adjustment reactions as pain duration increases and describes a series of developmental phases of chronic pain that he notes seem to parallel the responses to death and dying discussed by Kübler-Ross: denial, anger, bargaining, depression, and acceptance.[11,12] Fordyce describes the development of dysfunctional pain behaviors in terms of the individual's learning history.[9] Thus, a complex sequence of verbal and motor behaviors reflective of pain may be established via environmental reinforcement and come to dominate the individual's behavioral repertoire. In addition to overt pain behaviors, the development of negativistic and disabling patterns of thoughts and self-statements associated with pain has been identified by some authors as a hallmark of chronic pain.[13,14] Another approach views the transition of pain from acute to chronic in almost sociological terms, emphasizing the development of social roles and interactive patterns of illness behaviors that validate and unify perceptions of sickness and disability.[15,16,17]

An interesting concept to emerge from this sociological view of chronic pain is the term *pain career* proposed by psychologist Richard Sternbach.[18] This refers to the active, goal-directed behavior patterns of some patients with chronic pain. For such patients the order of the day is attention to medication and physical methods to relieve their pain, close monitoring of changes in their physical functioning, rigid adherence to patterns of rest and avoidance of physical activity, and interpersonal interactions devoted to discussion of their pain. Additionally, there may be considerable effort at resolving interminable legal issues associated with pain, including efforts to obtain disability ratings, struggles with insurance companies to underwrite medical care, or efforts to find better legal counsel to represent them. The above activities are suggestive of the career-like dedication of chronic sufferers to their pain and point out the necessity of altering not only specific pain behaviors but also focusing on the broader issue of the social and interpersonal contexts of these behaviors.

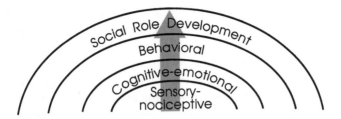

Figure 4.1 Developmental Stages of Pain: A Suggested Model

The above discussion, then, indicates that the meaning of pain tends to vary along a temporal dimension from a sensory signal of nociception to an increasingly unified sequence of emotions, cognitions, behaviors, and social roles. Figure 4.1 illustrates a suggested diagram of the sequential development of chronic pain. It is important to emphasize that considerable individual variation exists within and along this continuum and a given patient may very likely not exhibit all features described.

Stages of Pain: Empirical Evidence and Clinical Application

What evidence exists for the development of unique patterns of emotional reactions, behaviors, or social roles as pain progresses? What are the clinical implications of this for the clinician in the low back pain rehabilitation setting?

An early attempt to explore the psychological characteristics of chronic pain involved the administration of a widely used psychological test, the Minnesota Multiphasic Personality Inventory (MMPI), to a group of patients at varying stages of pain attending an orthopedic, low back pain clinic.[19] Of the total group of 117, 19 had pain of 6 months or less and were termed acute. The 98 patients with pain of 6 months or longer were termed chronic. The MMPI, based on responses to 565 true–false items, is interpreted with reference to the elevation of and pattern among thirteen psychometrically derived scales. Three of these scales are related to test-taking attitude and are termed *validity scales* and ten of the scales are reflective of psychopathological conditions and are termed *clinical scales*. Several interesting features emerged when the acute and chronic pain patients were compared. There was evidence of psychological reaction to pain in both groups. The acute patients revealed a tendency to deny emotions such as depression and to bolster this denial by a focus on symptoms of bodily distress which were reported in dramatic and magnified fashion. The acute patients also evidenced patterns of heightened cognitive and motor activity, perhaps reflecting efforts to cope with their recent pain onset. The chronic patients, in contrast, showed an even greater tendency to focus on physical complaints and symptoms, but appeared considerably less able to avoid unpleasant affects such as depression and relied less on pain coping strategies involving activity and anger. Thus, the study seemed to support the view that chronic pain patients are more depressed and somatically preoccupied, whereas acute pain patients are more anxious and agitated and appear to employ more active cognitive and motor coping strategies. These findings of increased focus on depression, somatic concerns, and symptom magnification in pain of increased chronicity have been corroborated in subsequent studies with both the MMPI and other assessment devices.[20,21] However, it is likely that this pattern is not only specific to chronic pain but may be seen in other chronic illnesses characterized by disruptions in activity and usual functioning.[20]

There is likewise empirical support for the emergence of a pattern of multiple dysfunctional behaviors as pain becomes more chronic and severe. A recent epidemiologic survey of 1016 patients in a health maintenance organization revealed that a large percentage (45%) of respondents noted some degree of recurrent pain problem.[22] However, only 1% reported pain over the previous 6 months that was persistent, severe, and associated with more than 7 disability days. The results also indicated that as pain becomes more persistent, severe, and disabling, patients reported increasing degrees of behavioral and social dysfunction, including increased health care visits, number of pain-related medications, and family stress. However, this and other studies have emphasized the increasingly individualized behavioral responses to pain as chronicity progresses and argued for personalized assessment of behavioral and emotional components in chronic pain.[23]

There are several implications of the acute–chronic pain distinction for the assessment and rehabilitation outcome of low back pain patients in the physical therapy setting. Frequently, physical therapists are accustomed to dealing with acute pain problems and tend to view pain primarily as an indication of tissue damage. The preceding section emphasizes the multiple components of chronic pain and the importance of assessing the affective, cognitive, and behavioral dimensions in addition to nociception. A discussion of useful assessment methods for the components of pain appears later in the chapter. The existing research, however, appears to caution against generic stereotypes of the chronic pain patient and suggests the need for individual assessment of each component of chronic pain. This should help to counter the frequent characterization of some patients with chronic pain as "crocks" or just needed to be motivated. Finally, the most important reason for distinguishing among the stages of pain is that interventions that are appropriate and even curative at one stage may aggravate and contribute to dysfunction at another. Table 4.1 illustrates this by contrasting management strategies that apply to earlier and later stages of pain.

Table 4.1 Management Strategies Appropriate to the Stages of Pain

Earlier Stages of Pain	Later Stages of Pain
1. Selective use of narcotics and muscle relaxants	1. Use of non-narcotic agents such as NSAI's
2. Selective use of immobilization	2. Increasing quotas of activity and re-conditioning exercises
3. Passive physical therapy modalities	3. Withdrawal of unnecessary prosthetic devices
4. Selective use of prosthetic appliances	4. Use of rest as a reinforcer for competent attainment of activity quotas
5. Use of pain as a signal to rest and to limit activity	

Disease versus Behavioral Models of Pain

As noted earlier, the view that pain is primarily an index of tissue damage has a long history and is useful for understanding pain as a biological survival system. This view can be described in general terms as part of the disease model in which pain is a symptom or signal of a pathophysiologic condition, often spatially distant from the site where it is perceived. In this model, the symptom of pain is primarily useful as an indicator of some underlying disease process elsewhere in the body. The treating clinician is often able to abolish or significantly dampen this sensory signal with medication or even surgical ablative procedures while attempting to modify the underlying pathology. We have seen, however, that as pain develops over time, a series of factors other than nociception comes to surround the experience of pain and that exclusive reliance on the disease model can be detrimental to patients with chronic pain. In short, the disease model fails to account for pain symptoms that are controlled by nonbiomedical factors, including current environmental influences and past learning history.

In contrast to the disease model, the behavioral model focuses on the myriad response alternatives that occur in the presence of physical symptoms. Although not writing directly about chronic pain, medical sociologist David Mechanic has been one of the major discussants on behavioral theories of illness, and he proposes the term *illness behavior* to describe the patient-determined response variables associated with any kind of medically defined disorder.[24] Mechanic notes that symptoms of any type are differentially evaluated, perceived, and acted on as a function of individual differences and social circumstances. He also makes the point, as yet rarely investigated in studies of people with pain, that a thorough understanding of the development of illness behavior requires the comparison of individuals who seek care for their symptoms with those who do not.

The insufficiency of the disease model when applied to the problem of pain is illustrated by a recent prospective study to identify risk factors for filing a back injury claim after a work accident.[25] Study participants included over 3,000 blue collar employees in a modern aircraft factory. During the 4-year study period, 279 employees filed injury claims. Other than a history of back problems, two psychosocial variables were found to be most predictive of those employees who reported symptoms: endorsement of an item indicating very low job satisfaction and high scores on Scale-3 (Hy) of the MMPI indicating a tendency toward somatic focus and symptom magnification. Thus, even for patients with acute pain in a sophisticated high-technology work setting, entrance into the health care system for the symptom of pain is determined by multiple factors not solely related to biomedical or disease variables.

The application of the behavioral model to chronic pain was a natural development in view of the gate control theory's emphasis on perceptual and reactive components of pain. The behavioral model focuses on the symptoms of pain in their varied observable features in addition to cognitive and environmental responses to them. Figure 4.2 contrasts these two models of pain. The disease model views pain as an external expression of underlying pathophysiological processes. The behavioral model emphasizes the centrality of the symptom of pain and stresses the multiple factors determining this symptom, including the environmental, cognitive, and nociceptive. In this section we examine two important clinical approaches derived from the behavioral model that are relevant to assessment: the environmental-operant approach and the cognitive-behavioral approach.

Environmental-Operant Approaches

Environmental-operant approaches to pain are based on the principle that behavior is determined by its environmental consequences. According to this principle, there is increased likelihood of a behavior occurring if it is followed by positive environmental effects and decreased likelihood of it occurring if there is either negative or no environmental effect. The rate of a behavior's occurrence is determined by the significance of the environmental reinforcement to the individual and the pattern in which the reinforcement is delivered. Thus, the strength of water as a reinforcer would increase as thirst increases and, generally speaking, once a behavior is acquired, its highest rate can be maintained by a variable schedule of reinforcement delivery, that is, reinforcement delivered after random numbers of responses or time sequences. These principles were most thoroughly inte-

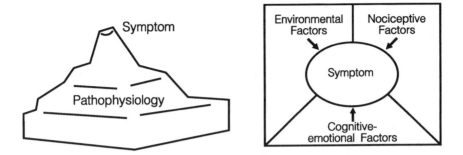

Figure 4.2 Disease Model (left) versus Behavioral Model of Pain

grated into American psychology through the work of B. F. Skinner. Their application to the evaluation and management of chronic pain was pioneered by the psychologist W. E. Fordyce[26] who has continued to advocate their application to a variety of chronic illnesses.[9] We will now examine the application of these concepts to the evaluation of pain.

Categories of Learned Behaviors

Psychologists recognize two major categories of learned behaviors—respondents and operants—and term the process of acquiring these behaviors *conditioning*. Respondent learning refers to behaviors that are elicited by antecedent stimulus conditions. Applied to pain behavior, respondent conditioning underlies those behaviors resulting from the antecedent condition of tissue injury or any other primary nociceptive process. For example, the patient who sustains a ruptured disc quickly learns to engage in the motor behaviors of guarding and bracing the musculoskeletal structures of the affected region and learns to avoid other motor behaviors that might elicit nociceptive input. Operant learning, on the other hand, refers to behaviors that are acquired and maintained as a consequence of their "operations" or effects on the environment. Much chronic pain behavior is acquired in this manner and is subject to the same principles of reinforcement governing any operant behavior.

Learned Acquisition of Pain

For a pain behavior to come under operant control, the reinforcement that follows it must be salient and must occur with some degree of frequency. Typically such environmental responses as attention or assistance from spouse, family members, or health care providers; drug use; rest;

or receipt of illness-related income may all act as powerful reinforcers for some pain patients. Thus, all varieties of pain behaviors, for example, bracing and grimacing, verbal complaints, motor inactivity, and even the use of prosthetic devices such as neck braces or canes, can be established and maintained by their environmental effects. Such behaviors are thus termed *pain operants*. It is important to note that behavior and behavior sequences can also be acquired through avoidance learning. That is, certain patterns of behavior are engaged in to avoid negative consequences. Much pain behavior such as excessive down time, guarding or bracing of body parts, or even avoidance of the work setting can be explained in this way.

Two points should be noted about this classification of learned behavior as applied to pain. One is that it is usually impossible to distinguish how a given behavior is acquired simply by observing it. That is, a limp resulting from a muscle sprain and one resulting from focused attention and solicitude by concerned family members may appear to be the same behavior. A second point is that often a behavior or behavioral sequence may be jointly determined by respondent and operant factors or may initially have been acquired via one mechanism and then maintained by another. These points underscore the fact that a behavioral evaluation of pain can be a complex task and argue against attempts at explaining all pain as a result of environmental conditioning. However, this should not deter the clinician from a careful assessment of the pain behaviors noted in individual patients along with the environmental responses to them from spouse, family members, and professionals. Also, a determination of what pain helps the patient to avoid is important via a question such as, "How would you be different if your pain could be totally relieved?" More will be said later in the chapter about structured methods for assessing behavioral components of pain.

Cognitive-Behavioral Approaches

In contrast to the environmental-operant model which focuses on observable, public behavior and external factors surrounding its acquisition and maintenance, the cognitive-behavioral model centers on covert, internal responses including thoughts, feelings, and patterns of coping with external demands. There has been a decided interest in recent years in the application of this approach to the assessment and treatment of patients with pain; typically, the focus is on the internal, self-directed statements patients make about their pain and their reactions to it.[14] In clinical pain practice, however, environmental-operant and cognitive-behavioral approaches are often employed concurrently to address the spectrum of behavioral factors in chronic pain that range from pain-contingent attention from family members and health care workers to dysfunctional self-reinforcement and coping skills in the patient.

Cognitive-Behavioral Assessment: General Strategies

Some primary assessment goals of the cognitive-behavioral approach are determination of perceived control over pain; perceived variation in intensity, frequency, and pattern of pain; and types of coping strategies employed to control pain. Patients are encouraged to write down thoughts and feelings associated with specific episodes of pain, and they are given training in reappraising these episodes via discussion with a cognitive therapist. Also, patients are trained in alternative strategies of coping with pain using such techniques as relaxation, attention-diversion, and rehearsal of responses to anticipated pain. Extensive literature exists on the application of these methods to chronic pain, and a psychometrically sound assessment tool, the Multidimensional Pain Inventory, has been devised to gather structured information on coping and affective responses to chronic pain.[27]

Cognitive-Behavioral Assessment:
Specific Applications for the Clinician

There are several assessment implications of the cognitive-behavioral approach for the clinician in the low back pain rehabilitation setting.

1. The clinician should observe and inquire about patients' attitudes toward pain. Do they appear overwhelmed, defeated, or challenged by pain? Is there a realistic, positive attitude toward achievement of rehabilitation goals or do patients insist on pain relief before engagement in rehabilitation? Is there a willingness to accept explanations offered for the etiology of the pain or do patients appear to be skeptical and ask for additional tests and evaluations? Do patients appear to be attending to information or instructions offered by the physical therapist? Can they repeat and demonstrate the instructions? Finally, do patients deny or underreport pain or set inappropriately ambitious rehabilitation goals for themselves?

2. The clinician should assess patients' perceptions of pain patterns and preferred strategies for coping with pain. When is the pain worse; when is it better? What effects do time of day, weather, season, activity, and rest have on pain? What can patients do to make the pain worse? To make it better? These questions help patients to recognize that pain is usually not constant and

unremitting but may have some predictable periodicity. Finally, patients can be encouraged to keep a daily diary of how they cope with episodes of pain and also times when pain is worst and least to help them anticipate ways of dealing with it.

3. The clinician should take an active role in supporting patients' use of appropriate coping strategies and assist them in acquiring additional ones, including progressive muscle relaxation, deep breathing, and distraction.

Techniques of Information Gathering in Clinical Pain Assessment

The following section surveys a variety of methods used to gather information on the components of pain. As emphasized throughout the chapter, pain is a complex phenomenon and accurate treatment planning requires individual assessment on the several dimensions of pain described earlier: nociceptive, environmental, and cognitive. The methods described are by no means inclusive of the wide array of techniques available for the assessment of pain. Nor is it necessary for the clinician to be able to employ all of the techniques described. The intent here is to assist the clinician in becoming an informed user/consumer of some of the more widely employed methods of assessment and also to enhance communication on this topic between the physical therapist and other members of the treatment team. Table 4.2 presents a summary of the techniques to be discussed.

Assessment Techniques Appropriate to the Nociceptive Component of Pain

Spontaneous Verbal Description of Pain

One universally employed technique is simply asking patients to describe their pain. Although this provides essential information in cases of acute pain, the data with chronic pain patients are more equivocal. For example, spontaneous verbal descriptions of pain have been reported not to distinguish organic from functional pain[28] and greater complexity of pain description has been found to be related to pain intensity.[29] However, other authors note more variable and diffuse pain descriptions in patients without organic disease.[30] Also, one study reported greater use of sensory descriptors (hot, burning) in nonorganic pain patients and use of affective descriptors (excruciating) in those with organic disease.[31] This would seem to suggest that simple reliance on spontaneous description of pain may have little diagnostic utility in *chronic* pain patients in addition to the likelihood that such descriptors may be affected by cultural factors.[32]

Table 4.2 Summary of Clinical Pain Assessment Techniques

Nociceptive Component
    Spontaneous verbal description of pain
    McGill Pain Questionnaire (MPQ)
    Visual Analog Scales (VAS)
    Physiologic assessment
    Pain maps

Cognitive-Reactive Component
    Clinical interview
      occupational history
      social history
    Psychological testing
      psychiatrically normed
      medically normed

Environmental Response Component
    Behavior ratings
      patient-based
      observer-based and automatic recording devices
    Information from spouse

McGill Pain Questionnaire (MPQ)

The McGill Pain Questionnaire (MPQ) was developed as a method for providing a standardized set of verbal descriptors for pain that could be compared across patients.[33] This instrument consists of adjectives grouped into three categories based on Melzack's theoretical distinction of three components of pain: sensory-discriminative, affective, and evaluative. The MPQ provides a number of scores based on the sum of scaled values for each word. These include scores for each of the three components of pain in addition to an overall score based on the total number of words chosen. This latter score has been shown to correlate with overall pain intensity.[34] Although the scale has been criticized for its length (a total of 78 adjectives contained in 20 categories), its difficulty for some patients, and statistical invalidity of its three-dimensional structure,[34,35,36] other studies have supported its factor structure[37] and noted satisfactory levels of reliability[38] and validity.[36] Recently, an improved method of scoring the MPQ to account for the uneven number of adjectives in each category has been reported.[39] The MPQ is probably one of the most widely used pain assessment methods and it has been translated into many languages. The data would seem to caution against simplistic reliance on classifying pain according to its three-dimensional structure, but it appears to be an excellent tool for establishing baseline levels of overall pain and for documenting treatment-related changes in pain perception.

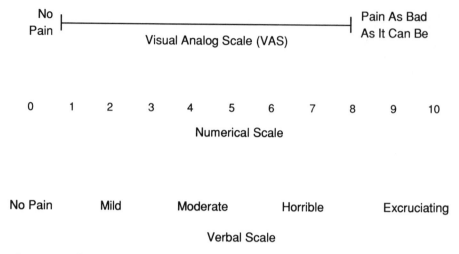

Figure 4.3 Three Types of Pain Rating Scales

Visual Analogue Scales (VAS)

The VAS is a commonly used method for globally evaluating pain. Typically, pain is rated on a scale of fixed length and the score is typically reported in centimeters. Line lengths of 10, 15, or 20 cm have been reported to be most reliable.[40] One study suggested that numbers not be imposed on the VAS due to preferential choice of certain numbers and that it be of a length that can be grasped as a unit, for example, 10 cm.[41] These authors also suggested that the VAS be administered initially in a supervised setting and advised the use of scale anchors such as severe, moderate, and slight, which extend over the length of the scale. In contrast to these specific recommendations regarding the format of the VAS, the use of other types and formats of rating scales has been described, including numerical scales and adjectival rating scales. Generally satisfactory correlations have been reported across these several types of rating scales, although patients are reported to express a preference for verbal scales.[42,43] It has also been suggested that patients with some impairment in abstraction, such as the highly medicated, the elderly, or those with a multisystem disease, respond most appropriately to numeric or adjectival-numeric scales.[43] Like the MPQ, the rating scale appears to be a simple method of documenting treatment-related changes in pain perception, but there is no convincing evidence to support the superiority of one rating scale method over another. Figure 4.3 provides three examples of pain rating scales.

Physiological Assessment

One assessment mode that frequently crosses professional discipline lines is that of physiological assessment. A frequent question is whether there are physiological characteristics unique to pain. Also, as biofeedback techniques become increasingly employed as a treatment approach for patients with pain, there is the question of physiological target and the specificity of the biofeedback training. For example, should biofeedback approaches be aimed at specific target muscle groups, or should they focus on more general goals such as reducing physiological arousal?

Earlier studies on the physiological effects of acute pain generally indicated a pattern of nonspecific physiological arousal responses roughly proportional to the intensity of the pain stimulus.[44] Such responses included increased heart rate, blood pressure, and striated muscle tension. In patients with chronic pain, however, there is little evidence for a linkage between physiological arousal and site or level of pain. More recent studies seem to support the earlier view of the lack of specific physiological patterns in patients with pain. For example, one study has shown that chronic low back pain patients do not differ from pain-free controls on levels of externally recorded EMG activity in back muscles during conditions of relaxation or stress;[45] nor do low back pain patients demonstrate differing patterns of autonomic arousal (heart rate, galvanic skin response) from pain-free controls.[46] A more promising direction appears to be looking at patterns of muscle activity, rather than the absolute levels of such activity, as there is some evidence for asymmetry in externally recorded EMG activity when the right and left sides of the back are compared in patients with low back pain.[47] Other studies have reported that postural factors, including prolonged standing, can amplify asymmetrical muscle activity and suggested serial bilateral assessments under differing patterns of activity.[48,49] However, there are no control studies allowing the conclusion that training patients to correct such muscle asymmetries will produce pain relief. One series of studies has reported that relaxation training is equally as effective as biofeedback in patients with chronic headache, leading the authors to speculate that symptom improvement may have resulted from anxiety reduction rather than specific physiological changes related to the biofeedback.[50]

The data thus argue against any specific physiological patterns unique to chronic pain. This must be balanced, however, against those individual cases where myofascial trigger points or zones of muscle spasm or hypertrophy appear to be correlated with pain episodes. It does appear in general that assessment of physiological parameters of anxiety and autonomic arousal, for example, heart rate, EMG activity in large striated muscle groups, or galvanic skin responses, may be of use in identifying those patients with chronic pain in whom anxiety may be contributing to symptom development or magnification.

Pain Maps

The use of pain maps or drawings on a figure of the human body for areas of experienced pain represents another assessment tool. In a sense this is a graphic analogue of the verbal reporting methods mentioned earlier. The pain map was used initially as a means of assessing anatomical accuracy of reported pain.[51] Later studies reported the development of a reliable method of scoring pain drawings,[52] and pain drawing scores have shown to correlate with the MPQ,[53] measures of psychopathology including symptom magnification and affective disturbance,[54] and pain-related disability.[55,56] Some authors have argued that the relationship between pain drawing scores and measures of pain intensity and frequency suggests that higher scores may reflect the "spreading of pain" phenomenon noted in myofascial pain syndromes (MPS).[55,56,57]

For the clinician in the low back pain rehabilitation setting, pain drawings represent a simply obtained measure of where the patient hurts. Reports of nondermatomal pain distribution can alert the therapist to possible psychological concomitants of pain, including depression, but may also reflect the wide distribution of pain found in MPS. The pain drawing would appear to represent a good marker for treatment effectiveness and could be administered serially during the rehabilitation process.

There is a cautionary note on the use of the pain map as well as the other nociceptive measures discussed in this section. All nociceptive measures require patients to attend to their pain and may thereby increase awareness of it. Also, the use of nociceptive measures may communicate an expectation to patients that a primary goal of treatment is relieving pain rather than the more realistic goal of improving function. Thus, nociceptive measures should be chosen judiciously, administered only when clinically appropriate, and combined with the other measures to be discussed in order to promote realistic treatment expectations to the patient.

Assessment Techniques Related to Cognitive-Reactive Component of Pain

This section describes a survey of several methods related to factors affecting patients' reactions to pain and the impact of pain on significant life functions.

Clinical Interview

The length and content of the clinical history taking in the rehabilitation setting is often determined by the interests of the professional discipline involved and the kinds of information needed by that discipline. The physical therapist is often engaged in assessment of the development of mechanical and activity limitations of the patient, but attention to the broader context and life impact of the pain through a brief interview can provide useful information.

Generally, it is best to begin by asking patients to describe their symptoms and the circumstances surrounding the onset of symptoms. Descriptions of the intensity, frequency, and patterning of pain are useful. The therapist should be attentive to the style of patients' responses in addition to the content. Are symptoms described in florid or dramatic terms? Do patients complain of severe, unremitting pain, yet appear comfortable and relaxed in the interview setting? A flat, unmodulated reporting style with little evidence of emotional or physical reactivity throughout the interview may provide evidence of depression. In contrast, anxious patients may evidence increased verbal and motor reactivity and display a worried concern over the meaning of their symptoms. Another item of interest is how the pain began. Some studies suggest that vague or unclear recollections about circumstances of onset or pain of exceptionally long duration should alert the clinician to evidence of cognitive impairment, possibly due to drug use or depression.[58,59] The therapist should also be alert to potential environmental issues surrounding the symptoms; for example, do symptoms prevent the patient from working or result in financial compensation? Did the symptoms begin in circumstances of anxiety or terror for the individual? Is the patient fearful of returning to a particular vocational or environmental setting? The author has seen a number of patients whose pain symptoms were coupled with a resulting post-traumatic stress disorder that significantly interfered with effective physical rehabilitation; for example, police or fire personnel injured in life-threatening circumstances, coal mining accidents or explosions, and motor vehicle accidents resulting in death or serious injury.

Although anxiety and depression are commonly observed as adjustment reactions to chronic pain, occasionally primary psychopathology may present in the context of a pain syndrome. Major depression, somatization disorder, hysterical conversion disorders, fictitious disorders, organic brain syndromes, and, rarely, psychotic disorders can all present with pain. The author recalls an undiagnosed paranoid schizophrenic who presented to the pain clinic with headache and who admitted after a brief interview that he believed the headaches were caused by an implanted radio transmitter. Although these cases would be relatively infrequent in the general chronic pain practice of the physical therapist, therapists should avail themselves of all existing medical history in addition to asking the patient about prior contacts with psychologists or psychiatrists.

Additionally, chronic pain syndromes may coexist in patients with other diagnosed mental or medical illnesses and this should not preclude such patients receiving treatment for their pain. In all such cases, consultation with a psychologist or psychiatrist with an interest in chronic pain is helpful.

Besides these obvious questions about the nature and context of the patient's symptoms, a brief social and occupational history is helpful for rehabilitation planning. Relevant social history includes marital status, family composition and living arrangements, recreational/vocational interests, spouse's occupation and reactions to the patient's symptoms, history of prior illnesses or pain-related illnesses in other family members, and history of prior or current physical or sexual abuse. This information will help to identify significant individuals in the patient's life who can help to reinforce treatment-related behaviors. Assessment of prior interests and activities can suggest behavioral outcome goals which can enhance the meaning of current treatment. Significant familial models of illness or a history of physical or sexual abuse can sometimes compromise rehabilitation and may indicate the need for psychological consultation. Occupational history items should include educational background; duration of present job and past job history; prior job-related injuries; satisfaction with job, employer, and coworkers; and willingness to consider job retraining. The above information gathered early in the rehabilitation process will aid the clinician in assessing the potential *disability* associated with the patient's symptoms and historical patterns predictive of future behavior, and suggest the need for potential involvement of other professionals including psychologists and vocational specialists.

Psychological Testing

Although the physical therapist will likely not be involved in the administration or interpretation of psychological tests in the rehabilitation setting, the following is a brief description of the application of psychological tests to patients with chronic pain.

Psychological test scores are based on the presentation, under standardized conditions, of a set of test items of known reliability and validity that are relevant to the psychological variable of interest. Individual test scores are compared to norms that are based on large numbers of responses to the test item by normal and various patient populations. Most psychological tests are easy to administer in any clinical setting and require only the ability to read and write English at a sixth-grade level. Some tests are available in languages other than English. For purposes of our discussion, the distinction can be made between psychological tests that have been developed and normed on patients with chronic pain or illness and those normed on other populations, typically psychiatric patients.

Generally speaking, tests that are developed and normed on chronic illness populations provide information on perception of illness, impact of illness on various areas of functioning, and preferred style of coping with illness. Tests of this sort that have received particular attention in the pain literature include: the Illness Behavior Questionnaire—a 52-item scale that provides scores on 7 scales relating to illness perception and psychological distress based on the previously discussed model of illness behavior by David Mechanic;[60] the Multidimensional Pain Inventory—a 61-item test providing scores on 13 scales reflecting the perception of the impact of pain on a broad array of life functions;[27] the Pain Locus of Control Scale—a 36-item scale that assesses the extent to which the patient explains control of pain in terms of personal resources, powerful others, or chance factors;[61] the Coping Strategy Questionnaire—a scale assessing the use of 42 strategies for coping with pain and ratings of perceived control of pain;[62] and the Millon Behavioral Health Inventory (MBHI)—a 150-item scale that provides scores on 20 dimensions relating to illness coping style, psychopathology, and psychosocial prognostic indicators.[63] The MBHI has been developed to be particularly useful to health providers, and the clinician may find it generates helpful ways of tailoring treatment strategies to psychological style. It may be ordered from the publisher mentioned in the reference.[63]

Perhaps the most widely used psychological instrument for pain assessment based on psychiatric norms is the MMPI. This test was described earlier along with its use to distinguish acute from chronic pain. As noted, MMPI profiles of chronic pain patients appear to be similar to those of patients with other chronic illnesses, with findings of increased depression, preoccupation with bodily symptoms, and a tendency to magnify symptom complaints. A more recent, and in some ways more clinically useful, application of the MMPI is to identify homogeneous subgroupings *within* the chronic pain population. A recent study described four clusters of MMPI scores ranging from extreme symptom magnification to normal and examined the relationship of cluster scores to treatment outcome.[64]

The preceding discussion emphasized the need for the clinician to appreciate the importance of cognitive style and symptom context in the response to pain. The use of interview and psychological test material, often obtained in collaboration with the clinical psychologist, can help to tailor the treatment plan to match preferred methods of coping and to set realistic goals for rehabilitation. A simple example would be the need to help "pace" the patient who responds to pain with anxiety and increased activity. This could be done by encouraging periods of rest after attainment of activity or exercise quotas. Additionally, factors such as fear of returning to a job, anger toward an employer or supervisor, litigation associated with personal injury or worker's compensation claims, or potential loss of social security or private disability payments can compromise rehabilitation goals and need to be assessed prior to embarking on a treatment regime.

Assessment Techniques Related to the Environmental Response Component of Pain

The significance of operant pain behaviors and the importance of evaluating the environmental consequences of pain were discussed earlier. The use of objective ratings of pain behavior can help to clarify the connections between such behavior and its environmental effects, including attention, rest, and avoidance of expected negative outcomes. Studies indicating little or no relationship between report of pain and activity level underscore the need for objective ratings of pain.[65]

Behavior Ratings by Patient

One approach is to have the patient record the amount of time spent in various categories of behavior on a daily basis. Fordyce suggests a diary type format, presented in Figures 4.4 and 4.5, for patient recording that includes time spent in the following behavior categories: sitting, walking, up-time, reclining, and don't know.[9] This format could be modified to include other behaviors relevant to specific rehabilitation goals. Patients are thus able to observe graphically their progress toward those goals in spite of fluctuations in levels of pain.

Behavior Ratings by Observers and Automatic Recording Devices

Another set of behavior recording methods involves recording by outside observers. These include scales that nursing personnel can employ in inpatient treatment settings[66] and interview rating scales.[67] Keefe has recently described a valid and reliable system for rating motor pain behaviors, including guarded movement, bracing, rubbing, grimacing, and sighing.[68] In addition, an automatic recording device has been developed that can be attached to the patient to record up-time.[69] Although up-time represents only a single category of behavior, one study found very low correlations between self-recording, observer-recording, and automated recording of this behavior.[70]

Spouse Information

One further source of information about the environmental effects of pain is the spouse or significant other. Even a brief interview with the spouse about the issue of responses to the patient's pain can prove helpful.

DAILY DIARY PAGE

Day of Week ————————————————

Date ————————————————————

Midnight	SITTING Major Activity	SITTING Time	WALKING Major Activity	WALKING Time	RECLINING Activity	RECLINING Time
12-1						
1-2						
2-3						
3-4						
4-5						
A.M. 5-6						
6-7						
8-9						
9-10						
10-11						
11-12						
NOON 12-1						
1-2						
2-3						
3-4						
4-5						
P.M. 5-6						
6-7						
8-9						
9-10						
10-11						
11-12						
TOTAL						= 24

Figure 4.4 Daily Diary Page (Reprinted with permission from Fordyce WE: Behavioral Methods for Chronic Pain and Illness. St. Louis, Mosby, 1976.)

DIARY ANALYSIS FORM

Name_____

Hosp. Number_____

Week in __ out__ No__	Sitting	Walking	Uptime	Reclining	Don't Know		Week in __ out__ No __	Sitting	Walking	Uptime	Reclining	Don't Know
TOTAL							TOTAL					
Avg/Day							x̄/Day					
Week in __ out__ No__	Sitting	Walking	Uptime	Reclining	Don't Know		Week in __ out__ No __	Sitting	Walking	Uptime	Reclining	Don't Know
TOTAL							TOTAL					

Figure 4.5 Diary Analysis Form (Reprinted with permission from Fordyce WE: Behavioral Methods for Chronic Pain and Illness. St. Louis, Mosby, 1976.)

Potential reinforcers of pain behavior include pain-contingent expression of solicitude and attention; caring for the patient's pain-related needs; and collaboration with the patient's avoidance of nonpain-related activities. The physical therapist is in an excellent position to engage the spouse as a therapeutic ally by encouraging positive responses to accomplishment of the patient's rehabilitation goals, increased time together in previously enjoyed activities, and disregard of inappropriate bids for attention related to pain complaints.

The material presented in this section encourages the clinician in the rehabilitation setting to assess treatment progress in ways other than pain relief. Indeed, helping the patient to see graphic increases on specific categories of behavior and eliminating environmental support for pain may significantly reduce the impact of pain in the patient's life.

It is important, however, to underscore the limitations of any self-report measure that can be influenced by mood states, cognitive factors, or environmental contingencies such as litigation or receipt of disability payments. Marked discrepancies in the patients's responses across the various components of assessment suggest the need for additional inquiry and discussion about these apparent inconsistencies. A simple example of this is the behavioral discrepancy noted in patients who complain verbally of excruciating, unremitting pain, yet display no motor or nonverbal evidence of pain. Of equal importance is the assessment of behavioral components of the physical therapy setting along with their contribution to rehabilitation outcome. Three simple examples of this are: (1) gradual elimination and withdrawal of unnecessary prosthetic devices which can trigger attention to pain by others in the patient's environment; (2) assessment of baseline activity levels for patients, including up-time, walking, and specific muscle strengthening activities; and (3) establishment of gradually increasing daily or weekly activity quotas using rest as a reinforcement for each activity cycle.

Conclusions

In summary, we have seen that the historical view of pain as a sensory system reflective of tissue damage has evolved into the present model which affords importance to the cognitive-reactive and environmental response components of pain. We have also looked at assessment methods for these components of pain with special relevance for the physical therapist in the low back pain rehabilitation setting. The intent of the chapter is to increase the clinician's familiarity with a broad range of assessment tools and to encourage their use as part of the regular evaluation procedure. Most of the approaches described require minimal time investment by the therapist and can have considerable benefit in terms of rehabilitation outcome.

Two points of general significance emerge from the material discussed. The first is the importance of sharing the assessment information with all members of the treatment team. No matter how thorough and elaborate the evaluation process, it will serve little purpose if the data is not communicated and viewed in the context of its treatment implications. This can sometimes be accomplished with a multidisciplinary staff conference where assessment data are pooled and a treatment plan is formulated. If this is not possible, the clinician should seek opportunities to integrate assessment information into the treatment plan. Furthermore, establishment of consultative relationships with other professionals, including psychologists, psychiatrists, and vocational therapists, can prove extremely valuable. This model emphasizes a collaborative, bidirectional communication flow among the rehabilitation professionals rather than the more traditional hierarchical medical model.

A second point of general significance is the importance of using assessment data as objective markers of individual patient and programmatic outcome. As indicated earlier, many of the assessment methods can be used to establish baselines from which future progress can be measured. The provision of such objective follow-up data is of great therapeutic importance to patients whose momentary perceptions of their status may be affected by transitory emotional or nociceptive factors. Likewise, the use of assessment data to document the overall effectiveness of the rehabilitation program is important for future program planning and to meet quality assurance criteria necessary for accreditation by national pain management boards such as the Committee for Accreditation of Rehabilitation Facilities (CARF). Physical therapists, because of their training in objective assessment and close contact with the patient, are in an ideal position to coordinate the overall evaluation of the patient on the components of pain that have been discussed. The hope is that this chapter will serve to encourage and catalyze that process.

References

1. Copp L: Pain and suffering. Am J Nurs 74:489–520, 1974.
2. Procacci P, Maresca M: A philosophical study on some words concerning pain. Pain 22:201–203, 1985.
3. Descartes R; L'homme. Paris, C Angot, 1664.
4. Melzack R, Wall PD: Pain mechanisms: A new theory. Science 150:971–979, 1965.

5. Bessou P, Perl ER: Responses of cutaneous sensory units with unmyelinated fibers to noxious stimuli. J Neurophysiol 32:1025–1043, 1969.

6. Payan DG: Neuropeptides and inflammation: The role of substance P. Annu Rev Med 40:341–352, 1989.

7. Hoffert M: The gate control theory re-revisited. J Pain Symptom Manage 1:39–41, 1986.

8. Melzack R, Wall P: The Challenge of Pain, rev ed. New York, Penguin, 1989.

9. Fordyce WE: Behavioral Methods for Chronic Pain and Illness. St. Louis, Mosby, 1976.

10. Merskey H (ed): Classification of chronic pain: Descriptions of chronic pain syndromes and definitions of pain terms. Pain (Suppl 3):S1–S225, 1986.

11. Hendler NH: The four stages of pain. In Hendler NH, Long DM, Wise TN (eds) Diagnosis and Treatment of Chronic Pain. Boston, John Wright, 1982.

12. Kübler-Ross E: On Death and Dying. New York, The MacMillan Co., 1969.

13. Lefebvre MF: Cognitive distortion and cognitive errors in depressed psychiatric and back pain patients. J Consult Clin Psychol 49:517–525, 1981.

14. Turk DC, Meichenbaum D, Genest M: Pain and Behavioral Medicine: A Cognitive-Behavioral Perspective. New York, Guilford Press, 1983.

15. Szasz TS: The psychology of persistent pain: A portrait of l'homme douloureux. In Soulairac A, Cahn J, Charpentier J (eds) Pain. New York, Academic Press, 1968.

16. Sternbach RA: Pain Patients; Traits and Treatment. New York, Academic Press, 1974.

17. Pilowsky I, Chapman CR, Bonica JJ: Pain, depression, and illness behavior in a pain clinic population. Pain 4:183–192, 1977.

18. Sternbach RA, Rustk TN: Alternatives to the pain career. Psychother Theory Res Pract 10:321–324, 1973.

19. Sternbach RA, Wolf SR, Murphy RW, Akeson WH: Traits of pain patients: The low-back "loser." Psychosomatics 14:226–229, 1973.

20. Naliboff BD, Cohen MJ, Yellen AN: Does the MMPI differentiate chronic illness from chronic pain? Pain 13:333–341, 1982.

21. Reading AE: A comparison of the McGill Pain Questionnaire in chronic and acute pain. Pain 13:185–192, 1982.

22. VonKorff M, Dworkin SF, LeResche L: Graded chronic pain status: An epidemiologic evaluation. Pain 40:279–291.

23. Zarkowska E, Philips HC: Recent onset vs. persistent pain: Evidence for a distinction. Pain 25:365–372, 1986.

24. Mechanic D: Medical Sociology, 2nd ed. New York, The Free Press, 1978.
25. Bigos SJ, Battie MC, Spengler DM, Fisher LD, Fordyce WE, Hansson TH, Nachemson AL, Wortley MD: A prospective study of work perceptions and psychosocial factors affecting the report of back injury. Spine 16:1–6, 1991.
26. Fordyce W, Fowler R, Lehmann J, Delateur B: Some implications of learning in problems of chronic pain. J Chronic Dis 21:179–190, 1968.
27. Kerns R, Turk D, Rudy T: The West-Haven Yale Multidimensional Pain Inventory (WHYMPI). Pain 23:345–356, 1985.
28. Klein RF, Brown WA: Pain descriptions in the medical setting. J Psychosom Res 10:367–372, 1967.
29. Boyd DB, Merskey H: A note on the description of pain and its causes. Pain 5:1–3, 1978.
30. Leavitt F, Garron DC: Psychological disturbance and pain report differences in both organic and non-organic low back pain patients. Pain 7:189–195, 1979.
31. Leavitt F, Garron DC, D'Angelo CM, McNeill TW: Low back pain in patients with and without demonstrable organic disease. Pain 6:191–200, 1979.
32. Zborowski M: People in Pain. San Francisco, Jossey-Bass, 1969.
33. Melzack R: The McGill Pain Questionnaire: Major properties and scoring methods. Pain 1:277–299, 1975.
34. Turk DC, Rudy TE, Salovey P: The McGill Pain Questionnaire reconsidered: Confirming the factor structure and examining appropriate uses. Pain 21:385–397, 1985.
35. Crockett DJ, Prkachin KM, Craig KD: Factors of the language of pain in patients and volunteer groups. Pain 4:175–182, 1977.
36. Reading AE: The internal structure of the McGill Pain Questionnaire in dysmenorrhoea patients. Pain 7:353–358, 1979.
37. Preito EJ, Hopson L, Bradley LA, Byrne M, Geisinger KF, Midax D, Marchisello PJ: The language of low back pain: Factor structure of the McGill Pain Questionnaire. Pain 8:11–19, 1980.
38. Hunter M, Phillips C, Rachman S: Memory for pain. Pain 6:35–46, 1979.
39. Melzack R, Katz J, Jeans ME: The role of compensation in chronic pain: Analysis using a new method of scoring the McGill Pain Questionnaire. Pain 23:101–112, 1985.
40. Revill SI, Robinson JO, Rosen M, Hogg MI: The reliability of a linear analogue scale for evaluating pain. Anaesthesia 31:1191–1198, 1976.
41. Scott J, Huskisson EC: Graphic representation of pain. Pain 2:175–184, 1976.
42. Downie WW, Leatham PA, Rhind WM, Wright V, Branco JA, Anderson JA: Studies with pain rating scale. Ann Rheum Dis 37:378–381, 1978.

43. Kremer E, Atkinson JH, Ignelzi RJ: Measurement of pain: Patient preference does not confound pain measurement. Pain 10:241–248, 1981.
44. Sternbach RA: Pain: A Psychophysiological Analysis. New York, Academic Press, 1968.
45. Nouwen A, Bush C: The relationship between paraspinal EMG and chronic low back pain. Pain 20:109–123, 1984.
46. Collins GA, Cohen MJ, Maliboff BD, Schandler SL: Comparative analysis of paraspinal and frontalis EMG, heart rate and skin conductance in chronic low back pain patients and normals to various postures and stress. Scand J Rehab Med 14:39–46, 1982.
47. Cram JR, Steger JC: EMG scanning in the diagnosis of chronic pain. Biofeedback and Self-Regul 8:229–241, 1983.
48. Hoyt WH, Hunt HH, DePouw MA, Bard D, Shaffer F, Passias JN, Robbins DH, Runyon DD, Semrad SE, Symonds JD, Watt KC: Electromyographic assessment of chronic low-back pain syndrome. J Am Osteopath Assoc 80:57–59, 1981.
49. Arena JG, Sherman RA, Bruno GM, Young TR: Electromyographic recordings of low back pain subjects and non-pain controls in six different positions: Effect of pain levels. Pain 45:23–28, 1991.
50. Blanchard EB, Andrasik F, Applebaum KA, Evans DD, Myers P, Barron KD: Three studies of the psychologic changes in chronic headache patients associated with biofeedback and relaxation therapies. Psychosom Med 48:73–83, 1986.
51. Ransford AO, Cairns D, Mooney V: The pain drawing as an aid to the psychologic evaluation of patients with low-back pain. Spine 1:127–134, 1976.
52. Margolis RB, Tait RC, Krause SJ: A rating system for use with patient pain drawings. Pain 24:57–65, 1986.
53. Toomey TC, Gover VF, Jones BN: Spatial distribution of pain: A descriptive characteristic of chronic pain. Pain 17:289–300, 1983.
54. Gill KM, Phillips G, Abrams MR, Williams DA: Pain drawings and sickle cell disease pain. Clin J Pain 6:105–109, 1990.
55. Tait RC, Chibnall JT, Margolis RB: Pain extent: Relations with psychological state, pain severity, pain history, and disability. Pain 41:295–301, 1990.
56. Toomey TC, Mann JD, Abashian S: Relationship of pain extent to ratings of pain description and function. Proceedings of the American Pain Society, 9th Annual Meeting, p. 28.
57. Travell JG, Simons DG: Myofascial Pain and Dysfunction: The Trigger Point Manual. Baltimore, Williams and Wilkins, 1983.
58. Swanson DW, Maruta T, Wolff VA: Ancient pain. Pain 25:383–387, 1986.
59. Hunter M, Philips C, Rachman S: Memory for pain. Pain 6:35–46, 1979.

60. Pilowsky I, Spence ND: Patterns of illness behavior in patients with intractable pain. J Psychosom Res 19:279–287, 1975.

61. Toomey TC, Mann JD, Abashian S, Thompson-Pope S: Relationship between perceived self-control of pain, pain description and functioning. Pain 45:129–133, 1991.

62. Rosenstiel AK, Keefe FJ: The use of coping strategies in chronic low back pain patients: Relationship to patient characteristics and current adjustment. Pain 17:33–44, 1983.

63. Millon T, Green CJ, Meagher RB: Millon Behavioral Health Inventory (MBHI). Minneapolis, National Computer Systems, Inc, 1981.

64. Costello RM, Hulsey TL, Schoenfeld LS, Ramamurthy S: P-A-I-N: A four-cluster MMPI typology for chronic pain. Pain 30:199–209, 1987.

65. Fordyce WE, Brena SF, Holcomb RJ, DeLateur BJ, Loeser JD: Relationship of patient semantic pain descriptions to physician diagnostic judgments, activity level measures and MMPI. Pain 5:293–303, 1978.

66. Swanson DW, Maruta T, Swenson WM: Results of behavior modification in the treatment of chronic pain. Psychosom Med 41:55–61, 1979.

67. Rybstein-Blinchick E: Effects of different cognitive strategies in the chronic pain experience. J Behav Med 2:93–102, 1979.

68. Keefe FJ, Hill RW: An objective approach to quantifying pain behavior and gait patterns in low back pain patients. Pain 21:153–161, 1985.

69. Sanders SH: Toward a practical instrument system for the automatic measurement of "up-time" in chronic pain patients. Pain 9:103–109, 1980.

70. Sanders SH: Assessment of up-time in chronic low back pain patients: Comparison between self-report and automated measurement systems. Paper presented at Association for Advancement of Behavior Therapy, New York, 1980.

5

Chronic Pain: Treatment Considerations

Philip W. Meilman

In chapter 4, assessment of the chronic pain patient was given extensive consideration. This chapter focuses on the treatment of that subset of chronic pain patients who have exhausted the standard medical and surgical treatment options, who are disabled by their pain, and whose pain is not caused by an active disease process. There are thousands of such patients, and they most commonly present with chronic back pain, often radiating into the extremities.[1,2] However, head-neck-and-shoulder pain and chronic headache complaints are not uncommon, and patients with unusual combinations of pain sites and even total body pain are sometimes encountered.

What makes these patients a challenge is the persistent nature of their pain and its intractability in the face of intensive efforts to treat it. As a result, the standard approaches to managing pain must eventually be relinquished in favor of methods that speak specifically to those particular issues presented by chronic pain patients.[3]

The standard methods of addressing pain are geared toward acute pain, that is, pain that is short-term in nature and that signals the presence of unhealed tissue damage. Rest, recuperation, and time away from physical pursuits are appropriate for acute situations, as are pain medications designed to relieve the patient of suffering. However, in the patients considered here, the tissues are mended and rest serves only to promote further deterioration of function; these patients have already been disabled for years.[4] Pain medications are not helpful and may in fact compound the problem by creating fatigue, lack of motivation, and addiction.[5]

Given this situation and the failure of traditional methods of treating pain, what can the clinician do? First, clinicians must reconceptualize the patient's situation as chronic and reconsider the basic treatment assumptions; second, they must have a coherent treatment plan; and third, that plan must then be translated into practice.

Basic Treatment Assumptions

The clinician must embrace several basic assumptions in working with this population.[6] The first is that the pain is real. This is critical. If there is any doubt in the physical therapist's mind, this will be communicated wittingly or unwittingly to the patient, and the patient will either become uncooperative or will go to great lengths to prove that the pain is real. Remember that the patient's credibility has likely been questioned already by treating physicians, friends, family members, and employers. Further questioning will serve only to alienate the clinician from the patient and may make the patient more difficult, if not impossible, to reach. In treatment, it is always important to accept the pain as real and never to question it.

Questions sometimes arise as to whether a patient is malingering. Most professionals working in the field agree that malingering is an extremely rare phenomenon.[7] A good working assumption is that patients are accurately representing their experience unless there is convincing evidence to the contrary—for example, a patient who cannot walk in the office but is observed walking on the street and is known to make more money on disability than when last employed.

A second important assumption is that the patient is not sick.[8] We know that this is the case because these patients have been through numerous evaluation protocols and have been diagnosed as not having an active or progressive disease process. Despite the disability and dramatic expressions of suffering, their pain is benign in origin. This knowledge enables us to approach the patient from a rehabilitation perspective. If there is any question in the physical therapist's mind as to the presence of an active disease process, then that issue needs to be clarified first. Likewise, patients need to accept the benign nature of their pain. If they raise a question as to whether another medical or surgical technique will help, this issue needs to be settled before attempting treatment. Otherwise, the patient will not fully invest in a rehabilitation-type program.

A third working assumption is that patients will be active participants in their own health care.[9,10] In traditional health care delivery systems, the patient is a passive recipient of services. However, it is precisely this passive orientation that contributes to the patient's expectation that health care personnel will magically cure him (an unlikely prospect) and that causes health care providers to do things "to" the patient (which do not help, either). While the traditional medical model generally works well in acute situations, such an approach is generally contrary to rehabilitation, and specifically to pain rehabilitation. Patients must take an active role in their own treatment. Ultimately, the patients' health is their own responsibility.[11]

Getting patients to this point requires considerable educational efforts, as patients are now being asked to take an approach that no other health care provider has previously requested of them. Therefore, the physical therapist will have to spend some time explaining the treatment philosophy and the need for the patients' active involvement. In doing this, it is helpful for the clinician to disavow any special healing powers and to let patients know that the potential for rehabilitation lies within themselves. The clinician might say, for example, "There is good news and bad news. The bad news is that I can't cure you. The good news is that I can teach you to do some things that can help you alleviate your own disability." If the new approach is further challenged, it may be helpful to say, "If the old ways of doing things had worked [meaning the passive, traditional approach], then you wouldn't be here right now. The fact that they haven't worked indicates that we must do things differently, and based on everything I know about chronic pain, this approach [active patient participation] is the right way to go."

A final assumption is that we are not actually treating pain at all; we are treating disability.[5] This notion may be confusing to the patient initially and may be confusing to the therapist if the therapist is unfamiliar with chronic pain management. However, this idea is central to the whole process. If therapists imply or state that they are treating pain, patients will be on the lookout for pain relief. Paradoxically, this attention to pain relief as the measure of success almost insures that it will not happen. This occurs because the focus is on the pain. The more a patient focuses on pain, the more central, important, and noticeable it becomes. Instead, the focus of treatment must be the alleviation of disability. This is far more attainable and objectively measurable. Clinical experience has shown that if pain relief is to occur at all, it will happen after the disability is eliminated, not before. And even if pain is not eliminated, if the disability can be eliminated, then the pain is of little functional consequence and thus recedes in importance.

Getting this idea across to the patient is vital, and it is helpful to be explicit. The clinician could say, for example, "You have a chronic pain syndrome, and you have had it for many years. Most people with chronic pain accept their disability but fail to accept the pain, putting their lives on 'hold' while they wait for the pain to go away. I need to teach you that the way to manage this problem is to reverse your stance: you need to accept the pain but not the disability." And then the clinician could add, "You need to know that you may have pain for the rest of your life. That's the nature of chronic pain. Some days it's sharp and shooting, some days it's dull and throbbing, some days it's to the left, some days to the right, some days it's good, other days it's bad. This may stay with you. But you don't need to be disabled by pain. You can work toward walking normally again, you can work toward handling your responsibilities again, you can work toward playing with your kids again. And the interesting part is that when you fully overcome your disability, you may find that your pain becomes less important or unimportant; a few lucky patients even report that it goes away—but this happens only after the disability is alleviated, not before, and it can't be guaranteed. The most important thing is for you to get on with your life, pain or no pain. And that's what I'm here to help you accomplish."

Treatment

Treatment itself can be divided into three general areas: medication withdrawal, interventions for psychological and attitudinal issues, and physical rehabilitation.

Medication Withdrawal

With respect to medication withdrawal, it must be understood that most benign, chronic, disabled pain patients are addicted to their pain medications.[12,13] Benzodiazepines are sometimes prescribed as "muscle relaxants," whereas narcotics and barbiturates are often prescribed specifically for pain relief. Sleeping pills may also be prescribed. All of these medications are highly addictive. It is not uncommon for pain patients to take their medications in excess of the prescribed doses. Even if these drugs are taken in the prescribed manner, the prescription may have been inappropriately continued for years, in spite of the fact that most pain medications are intended for short-term use. When patients take these medications over a period of months and years, they develop an increasing tolerance to the effects and need ever-increasing doses to obtain the same relief. As they continue to pour quantities of sedating and tranquilizing drugs into their systems, they become lethargic, fatigued, distracted, and unmotivated, and they experience memory and concentration difficulties. Since chronic pain rehabilitation requires motivation and an investment of energy, the use of pain medications runs directly counter to the goals of treatment.

Weaning patients from their medications should be done in the context of a pain rehabilitation program that offers them alternative coping methods. Otherwise, they may experience a sense of loss and panic as their medications are withdrawn. Assuming that medication withdrawal is done in this context, then the tried-and-true method is to gradually taper patients from what they have been taking before entering treatment and then slowly reduce and then eliminate their medications altogether.[3] Often the medications are disguised in nondescript capsules or sweet-tasting "pain cocktails" to avoid the problem of patients focusing on dosages and their assumed relation to pain levels.[2] Three to four weeks is generally sufficient time to complete a medication withdrawal protocol. Drugs used for other medical conditions, such as antihypertensives, are not included in the protocol.

Comprehensive inpatient or day treatment programs almost always include medication withdrawal as part of the treatment plan. On the other hand, the independent practitioner, treating chronic pain patients individually, will need to work closely with a physician with whom there is a shared understanding of the need for medication withdrawal and an agreed-on protocol to accomplish this. A good working relationship with a physician knowledgeable about chronic pain rehabilitation is important. The physical therapist can then attend to the physical side of the program, comfortable in the knowledge that the medication is gradually being reduced and ultimately eliminated.

Clinical experience has shown that dependence on pain medications is usually secondary to the pain problem. Once the patient is rehabilitated, the medication issue becomes less problematic. However, there is a subset of these patients, about 20% according to one study,[12] who have a primary addiction to these drugs and who may need treatment for chemical dependency after completing a pain program;[14] otherwise, they will not be able to keep themselves free of medication. All patients, however, must be forewarned about the temptation to turn to pills when attempting to cope with a "bad" day after treatment is completed. Bad days are inevitable, and patients need to be encouraged to exercise, talk with someone, or otherwise distract themselves from reaching into the medicine chest. Taking one pill may not be harmful in itself, but that makes it easier to take a second, and the second makes it easier to take a third, and so on. Thus, a medication dependency can easily be reestablished.

Health care personnel who are trained to listen for and recognize the denial process present in alcoholism and other drug dependencies can be helpful in assessing the patient's status.[15] A patient's family is also a good source of information as the patient engages in treatment. If a patient has a primary addiction, then a long-term plan for intervention and rehabilitation should be arranged. Even if a patient does not have a primary addiction, individual and group discussions regarding the nature of mood-altering drugs, tolerance, loss of control, withdrawal, and craving can be helpful in the treatment process. Films and presentations by substance abuse professionals and by recovering alcoholics or addicts can also be helpful.

Of course, a clinician's being knowledgeable about medications is no protection against being fooled by patients who disguise their unauthorized use.

This can and does happen, and most professionals who have worked closely with chronic pain patients can recount instances where they have been deceived by a patient who was using drugs surreptitiously. A dramatic example is the elderly woman, a prototypically sweet grandmother type, who kept vodka in her hand lotion bottles while an inpatient on a chronic pain treatment unit. She had also been ordering Librium for years on her husband's veterinary license without his knowledge. So it can and does happen even to those who are skilled in this area.

Some workers in the field routinely prescribe antidepressants for chronic pain patients based on assumptions that antidepressants have an analgesic effect or a sleep-enhancing effect or that pain is a "depressive equivalent."[16] However, in most cases, this is not necessary. As patients are remobilized, the depression that may have been evident on their initial presentation may lift spontaneously as they see themselves becoming increasingly more competent and functional. However, there may be some cases where antidepressants are useful, and here again, it is helpful to establish a working relationship with a physician who understands chronic pain management.

Psychosocial Issues

Psychosocial issues are a second major treatment concern in chronic pain rehabilitation. These issues can be further divided into attitudinal factors and psychological factors.

Attitudinal Factors

With respect to attitude, there are several important points to consider. First, the patient needs to have an accepting attitude toward the treatment philosophy. The patient must have relinquished the hope that a medical or surgical approach will provide the "magic bullet" that will cure the pain if this approach is to work. As long as patients hold out hope that there is another pill or another surgery or another technique that will cure them, they will always be questioning the wisdom of the approach and will always be looking over their shoulder for another pain-relieving technique. This seriously compromises the ability of the physical therapist or any members of the treatment team to have an impact.

Patients who are appropriate for chronic pain management techniques need to be given a consistent and unequivocal message by their physicians and their physical therapists that they will not injure themselves by participating in a rehabilitation program, that they will not paralyze themselves, and that they will not "rupture their discs." Such unspoken fears may indeed be present if they are not directly addressed, and this will adversely affect the patient's ability to invest in the treatment.

Attitude can also be affected by the presence of ongoing litigation. Pain patients may have pending litigation for any number of purposes—for recovery of medical expenses, for lost wages, for pain and suffering, to express anger, or for combinations of these factors.[17] At the same time, patients may have varying degrees of investment in the litigation process. Some are highly invested; others leave it up to their attorneys and are not emotionally invested in what happens.

Those who are invested in their lawsuits present a more difficult treatment situation because their ability to participate in a rehabilitation program may be adversely affected.[18] Some chronic pain treatment programs do not accept patients with pending litigation and some accept them only if the attorney can provide assurances that the outcome of litigation will not depend on the outcome of treatment.[19,20] Other programs accept patients with pending litigations and work with them to reduce their preoccupation with legal issues. This is an important undertaking because of the clinical finding that as the date of court hearings approaches, patients become distracted and obsessed with the outcome or with perceived injustices that the hearing is meant to address. These patients then deteriorate as the court date approaches.[18] Thus, it is important to assess patients' concerns about litigation in an ongoing fashion during the course of treatment and to work with patients around the need to make rehabilitation, and not lawsuits, their most important job. Discussions regarding the possible realistic outcomes and the contrast with imagined "pie in the sky" settlements are important. Of course, there *are* some dramatic settlement awards, but these are rare occurrences. Most settlements do not provide vast sources of wealth, and in fact many of them are quite meager. When patients are apprised of this, it helps change attitudes about litigation.

Potential for reemployment also greatly affects attitude. If someone is assured of employment upon successful rehabilitation, this is—for most people—more motivational than when employment possibilities are unknown. The contribution of an employment counselor or rehabilitation worker can be a great asset to a pain program. This professional can also provide input into a work hardening program designed by the physical or occupational therapist.

Another important aspect of treatment involves teaching the patient a "can do" attitude—an attitude in which the patient can say, "I am going to get on with my life, pain or no pain." Previously, pain had been the reason for engaging or not engaging in activities. For these patients, life has been put on "hold" for many years, typically, while the pain persists. The new attitude that needs to be inculcated is that life cannot be made contingent on pain. As we have said repeatedly to patients, it is the difference between saying, "I'm going to go out Saturday night if I feel good," and saying, "I'm going to go out

Saturday night," and then following through. In the first case, plans are contingent on pain; in the second case, there is a firm commitment. Thus, in this prototypical way, personal goals can supplant pain with respect to decision making.

Psychological Factors

Individual psychological factors can be assessed and addressed in a comprehensive approach that includes mental health personnel (usually psychologists) in addition to physical therapists, physicians, nurses, and occupational therapists. As treatment progresses, the patient's "story" unfolds, and the psychological issues become more apparent.

Where a comprehensive team approach is not practical, it may be somewhat harder to discern individual psychological factors because information cannot be gathered as quickly or as comprehensively, but it is still possible to gather this important data. For this purpose, it may be useful to team up with a psychologist who is knowledgeable about treatment approaches for chronic pain. Presenting the psychologist as someone who can teach patients and their families new ways to cope with pain and stress and thus accelerate the rehabilitation process may well convince reluctant patients to accept a consultation. In looking for a psychologist, it is important to seek out someone who is skilled in rehabilitation approaches rather than a general psychotherapist. Ideally, the psychologist should have a background in chronic pain treatment and behavioral medicine techniques.

With respect to psychological factors in chronic pain, it is important to remember that initially these patients present in remarkably similar ways. Their distress, they say, is secondary to their pain, and if the pain could only be relieved, then all of their problems would be alleviated—marital difficulties, depression, work-related problems, sexual dysfunction, financial concerns, lack of mobility.[21] As they work on rehabilitation, however, the issues peculiar to their individual situations begin to stand out in bold relief. For example, one headache patient with extraordinarily tight neck and shoulder muscles discovered on the inpatient treatment unit that her muscle tension was related to an inability to be assertive. Instead of talking about her needs, she would bottle up her concerns, unconsciously tighten up her musculature, and then develop headaches. Furthermore, this happened almost all the time at home. Another patient, a middle-aged man, was greatly distressed about his grown children's welfare, and burst into tears in a torrent of previously unexpressed emotion within the safety of the psychologist's office. He had never before discussed his worries, and these were clearly related to his overall state of tension, which of course impacted on his pain. Counseling could then be effectively directed to his family issues.

It is important for regular and frequent meetings to take place between patients and the treating mental health professionals during the course of pain rehabilitation to keep abreast of issues that surface as patients work their way through the program. Issues arise often, especially early in the treatment, and they need to be addressed as they occur. Otherwise, they tend to interfere with the patient's progress.

Family involvement in treatment is important to the patient's progress and to treatment outcome.[22,23] Families need to learn how to care for the patient without catering to or caring for the pain. Because this approach runs counter to what common sense and ordinary logic suggest that one should do for a patient who is ill, families will need direct instruction and guidance. Instead of fetching items or running errands for patients, families need to encourage patients to do for themselves. If the patient is having a bad day, the family's new response should be, "Let's go out for a walk," or, "Let's do some exercises," rather than, "'Why don't you lie down and rest. I'll do the dishes." This is a challenge, and families will need support in carrying this out—and they will need to be monitored. With some fine tuning, most families are able to follow these directions. Some families are highly resistant to this, however, and this tells us something about their degree of investment in the pain problem and the complex nature of their family dynamics.

For most families, however, helping the pain patient get better is paramount, and they will be receptive. It also helps to address with families the disappointment, anger, fear, apprehension, and miscommunication that have resulted from the chronic pain syndrome. Further, spouses need to address the sexual dysfunction or loss of interest that almost always occurs in chronic pain situations and which, in turn, adversely affects the marital relationship.

Stress management and biofeedback are often considered important aspects of pain management. In a general sense this is true. However, neither stress management nor biofeedback should be held out to the patient as pain-relieving techniques. If such a representation is made or implied, the patient may view these as potential "magic bullets" that will take the pain away. Thus, false expectations are created that run counter to the treatment philosophy and leave the patient feeling disappointed when pain relief is not forthcoming. Instead, biofeedback and stress management should be presented as tension reduction methods and as ways to achieve a healthier lifestyle; ideally, patients have already been exposed to the concept that pain causes considerable tension and stress, and so they will understand that these techniques can create that healthier lifestyle they so desperately need.[24]

Some time needs to be devoted to teaching patients how to recognize stressors in their lives and how to identify their idiosyncratic reactions to those stressors. If a situation with an employer causes tension, for example, environmental manipulations can be made to reduce tension—such as minimizing contact with the boss—and cognitive techniques can reduce tension as well—for example, labelling the boss as someone who is stressed rather than as someone who is dictatorial. Another "cognitive" stress reduction technique involves examining one's style of information processing and adjusting it when it leads to unrealistic conclusions.[25] For example, if a patient routinely "catastrophizes," or imagines the worst possible outcomes in any given situation, this will keep stress levels and muscle tension high. Thus, if a patient routinely imagines that his wife has been in an auto accident whenever she does not arrive home on time, this will markedly increase his stress. The ability to identify such troublesome thinking patterns and substitute more realistic appraisals can significantly lower emotional distress and muscle tension.

Formal tension reduction techniques, such as diaphragmatic breathing and deep muscle relaxation, can also be taught as ways to reduce a patient's overall level of arousal.[26] Relaxation techniques need to be practiced and used several times a day to have a good effect. Sporadic use is largely ineffective, as is an isolated application at a time of high anxiety. Again, these techniques should be presented as one way of creating a healthier lifestyle rather than as pain-relieving techniques.

Physical Therapy

The physical side of treatment is, of course, of most concern to the physical therapist. Specific exercise programs and lists of exercises are available from a variety of sources.[27,28] However, this section reviews some aspects of the philosophy of treatment because the physical therapy techniques that are used will flow from that philosophy.

As noted earlier, decisions about function can no longer be based on pain once a patient enters treatment. In other words, the patient, with the assistance of treatment staff, must now formulate physical as well as personal goals and must gradually work toward those goals in a consistent manner. This means that pain can no longer be the relevant variable in physical therapy; the long-term exercise goals and daily subgoals are now the important factors. "Working to tolerance" is no longer appropriate; working to criterion is the important factor. In support of this, there is evidence to suggest that pain complaints either remain the same or decrease with activity in these patients.[29,30]

As an example of working to criterion, let us assume that the patient wants to be able to exercise on a bicycle 20 minutes, 3 times a day. However, his baseline ability is only 2 minutes per session. On Day 1, the patient can start at his baseline level 3 times per day. Then he can increase his time by one minute—a barely perceptible increase. Thus, on Day 2, he is riding the exercycle 3 minutes, 3 times per day. On Day 3, he rides the exercycle 4 minutes, 3 times per day; and so on for each succeeding day. Once he has reached his goal of 20 minutes, 3 times per day, he maintains at that level. A similar approach can be used for walking, stairclimbing, and other forms of exercise.

The key here is to teach the patient that if he has a "good" day, he should not exceed his subgoal for that day. Similarly, if he has a "bad" day, he should not relinquish his subgoal for that day, either. Pain patients universally report good days and bad days, but effective pain rehabilitation means functioning up to criterion, regardless of the kind of day it is.[31] Thus, the treatment program is designed to increase stamina, endurance, and tolerance and to develop an attitude of functioning even when pain is present.

Patients will not ordinarily recognize their progress from one day to the next, nor from one week to the next, nor from one month to the next. This can be demoralizing, with a consequent negative effect on morale and motivation. To prevent this from happening and provide the patient with positive feedback on his progress, the use of charts and graphs is recommended for each targeted goal.[27] The patient will likely be keeping a large number of graphs—one for each exercise and activity—but this is most useful and provides the patient with a clear sense of progress. If the patient is truly following the program, the graphs should look like stairsteps leading up to a landing, which represents the maintenance level. Work hardening programs can follow this same general plan, with the workload gradually increasing until the final goal is reached. Measures of spinal range of motion (for example, gross lumbar range, true lumbar range, straight leg raising) can also help assess progress,[32] and the results can be charted along with other records of exercise.

A maintenance program is important long after the formal pain rehabilitation program is finished. Patients need to know that they must continue on an exercise program for the rest of their lives. While individuals without chronic pain ideally should be on an exercise program too, they can generally survive without one. This is not the case for chronic pain patients, however. Without exercise, their muscles, tendons, and ligaments are likely to shorten, tighten, and become less flexible, a situation they can ill afford.

In this rehabilitation approach, the physical program largely involves work done by the patient under the supervision of the therapist. There is a role, of course, for the physical therapist to use manual therapy and other "passive" techniques on patients, but these are most appropriate at the beginning of treatment, and the patient can be weaned from them as treatment progresses. In addition, whirlpool and massage—often used as treatments themselves in other settings—are excellent rewards for a patient's performing an exercise program up to daily subgoals, instead of being defined as "treatments" for chronic pain.

As part of therapy, the entire treatment team, and especially the physical therapist, needs to identify "pain behaviors."[31,33] These are actions that signal to the world that the patient does not feel well, including limping, leaning, guarding, moaning, saying "I can't," and lying down. Pain behaviors are sometimes subtle and sometimes not-so-subtle forms of communication that create expectations of disability for both patient and audience. Pain behaviors keep the patient focused on the pain and perpetuate the disability. Effective chronic pain management entails helping patients identify their pain behaviors and then working with them to eliminate these forms of communication.

When the physical therapist recognizes and rewards the elimination of pain behaviors and notices positive gains, it is quite motivating for the patient. As pain behaviors decrease, the physical therapist can teach techniques of good body mechanics, which can then be substituted for the pain behaviors.

In settings where there is a critical mass of patients in treatment, group feedback as to patients' progress (or lack thereof) can be especially useful.[34] Chronic pain patients are often difficult to work with, and they occasionally set up a "we-they" antiauthority stance with treatment staff. To mitigate this, the use of feedback from fellow patients as well as staff is often helpful. It is far more powerful for one pain patient to say to another, "You are cutting corners on your exercise program," or, "You are demonstrating more pain behavior this week than last week," than it is for the physical therapist to give the same input, although that is important, too.[35] Patients can be confrontive, supportive, and encouraging with each other in a way that has significant impact and therapeutic effect. A compliment from one pain patient to another about a good effort, or a shared concern about difficulties that lie ahead, can be most therapeutic. By way of suggestion, it is helpful to call these meetings "group feedback" sessions or "weekly performance reviews." Calling it group therapy may send patients scurrying in other directions.

Conclusion

It should be evident from this discussion that the treatment of chronic pain is complex and that doing it well requires coordination of efforts. Professionals working in strict isolation cannot provide the kind of therapeutic environment or treatment coverage needed. Therefore, before attempting to provide services for chronic pain patients, a treatment team or a consulting group should be formed and a therapy program developed. When this is done well, it is of great service to chronic pain patients.

Sometimes, though, even the best of efforts do not work and the patient remains debilitated and/or maintains a negative attitude toward treatment. If such is the case, it may be helpful to refer the patient to a chronic pain inpatient or intensive day hospital program. Often, these 4- to 6-week programs are housed in university-based hospitals or major rehabilitation facilities. The intensity of services maximizes the chance of patients getting better, although even then, not all will do well. For example, in a well-controlled study, Guck et al. found that 60% of patients were successful (as defined by strict criteria) on a 1- to 5-year follow-up, as compared with 0% of matched controls who did not have treatment. But this still left 40% who were not classified as complete successes. Some were partially helped and some were not helped at all.[36] So clinicians need to remember that they will not always be successful, even when they give it the best effort possible.

References

1. Sternbach RA: Pain Patients: Traits and Treatment. Orlando, Academic Press, 1974.
2. Fordyce WE: Behavioral Methods for Chronic Pain and Illness. St. Louis, Mosby, 1976.
3. Turk DC, Meichenbaum D, Genest M: Pain and Behavioral Medicine. New York, Guilford Press, 1983.
4. Weisenberg M: Pain and pain control. Psychological Bulletin 84:1008–1044, 1977.
5. Fordyce WE, Steger JC: Chronic pain. In Pomerlau OF and Brady JP (eds) Behavioral Medicine: Theory and Practice. Baltimore, Williams and Wilkins, 1979, pp. 125–153.
6. Meilman PW: Chronic pain: Basic assumptions regarding treatment. Journal of Orthopaedic and Sports Physical Therapy 5:308–310, 1984.
7. Leavitt F, Sweet JJ: Characteristics and frequency of malingering among patients with low back pain. Pain 25:357–364, 1986.
8. Pinsky JJ, Crue BL, Griffin S: Why a pain unit? In Crue BL (ed) Chronic Pain: Further Observations from the City of Hope National Medical Center. New York, SP Medical and Scientific Books, 361–372, 1979.
9. Finer B: Treatment in an interdisciplinary pain clinic. In Barber J and Adrian C (eds) Psychological Approaches to the Management of Pain. New York, Brunner/Mazel, 186–204, 1982.
10. Pinsky JJ, Malyon AK: The intractable pain and suffering process: Facilitating change. In Crue BL (ed) Chronic Pain: Further Observations from the City of Hope National Medical Center. New York, SP Medical and Scientific Books, 315–320, 1979.

11. Swanson DW, Swenson WM, Maruta T, McPhee MC: Program for managing chronic pain. I. Program description and characteristics of patients. Mayo Clin Proc 51:401–411, 1976.

12. Davis JC: Analgesic and psychoactive drugs in the chronic pain patient. Journal of Orthopaedic and Sports Physical Therapy 5:315–317, 1984.

13. Maruta T, Swanson D, Finlayson R: Drug abuse and dependency in patients with chronic pain. Mayo Clin Proc 54:241–244, 1979.

14. Florence D: Chronic pain: Fact or fiction. Minn Med 63:781–782, 1980.

15. Meilman PW, Gaylor MS: Substance abuse. In Grayson PA and Cauley K (eds) College Psychotherapy. New York, Guilford Press, 1989, pp. 193–215.

16. Blumer D, Heilbronn M: Chronic pain as a variant of depressive disease: The pain-prone disorder. Journal of Nervous and Mental Diseases 170:381–406, 1982.

17. Meilman PW: On the difficulties of coding pain-related data. Pain 36:133–134, 1989.

18. Meilman PW: Chronic benign pain syndromes: Questions commonly asked by attorneys. Westchester Bar Journal 15:223–230, 1988.

19. Roberts AH: The Pain Clinic and Pain Treatment Program Procedure Manual. Minneapolis, University of Minnesota Hospitals, 1975, unpublished manuscript.

20. Sternbach RA, Wolf SR, Murphy RW, Akeson WH: Traits of pain patients: The low-back "loser." Psychosomatics 14:226–229, 1973.

21. Meilman PW: Psychological aspects of chronic pain. Journal of Orthopaedic and Sports Physical Therapy 1:76–82, 1979.

22. Dunbar J: Adhering to medical advice: A review. International Journal of Mental Health 9:70–87, 1980.

23. Baekeland F, Lundwall L: Dropping out of treatment: A critical review. Psychological Bulletin 82:738–783, 1975.

24. Guck TP: Stress management for chronic pain patients. Journal of Orthopaedic and Sports Physical Therapy 6:5–7, 1984.

25. McKay M, Davis M, Fanning P: Thoughts and Feelings: The Art of Cognitive Stress Intervention. Richmond, CA, New Harbinger Publications, 17–45, 1981.

26. Armentrout DP: A holistic approach to treating chronic pain. Paper presented at the Second World Congress on Pain, Montreal, Canada, August 1978.

27. Siracusano G: The physical therapist's use of exercise in the treatment of chronic pain. Journal of Orthopaedic and Sports Physical Therapy 6:73–88, 1984.

28. Percival J, Percival L, Taylor J: The Complete Guide to Total Fitness. Ontario, Prentice Hall of Canada, 1977.

29. Linton SJ: The relationship between activity and chronic back pain. Pain 21:289–294, 1985.
30. Fordyce W, McMahon R, Rainwater G, Jackins S, Questad K, Murphy T, De Lateur B: Pain-complaint-exercise performance relationship in chronic pain. Pain 10:311–321, 1981.
31. Meilman PW: Legitimizing chronic pain. Journal of Orthopaedic and Sports Physical Therapy 5:312–315, 1984.
32. Mayer TG, Gatchel RJ, Kishino N, Keeley J, Capra P, Mayer H, Barnett J, Mooney V: Objective assessment of spine function following industrial injury: A prospective study with comparison group and one-year follow-up. Spine 10, 482–493, 1985.
33. Fordyce WE: Behavioral Methods for Chronic Pain and Illness. St. Louis, Mosby, 1976.
34. Gottlieb H, Strite LC, Koller R, Madorsky A, Hockersmith V, Kleeman M, Wagner J: Comprehensive rehabilitation of patients having chronic low back pain. Archives of Physical Medicine and Rehabilitation 58:101–108, 1977.
35. Sternbach RA: Varieties of pain games. In Bonica JJ (ed) Advances in Neurology (Vol. 4), New York, Raven Press, 1974.
36. Guck TP, Skultety FM, Meilman PW, Dowd ET: Multidisciplinary pain center follow-up study: Evaluation with a no-treatment control group. Pain 21:295–306, 1985.

6

□ □ □
□ □ □
□ □ □

Managing Symptom Magnification

Robert B. King

Editor's Note: The information contained in this chapter is the product of careful observation, patient interactions, interactions with multiple professionals, and a solid clinical background spanning more than 20 years. Like chapter 8, this chapter is empirically based, fairly representing the "state of the art" in this area. Much of the chapter is written in the first person, reflecting the author's style and reminding the reader of the empirical nature of the material. To date, only a few controlled studies have examined management of patients exhibiting symptom magnification behaviors. The information contained within the pages of this chapter should serve as a source of lively discussion, humorous anecdotes about experiences with our own patients, and practical information that can help the reader today in the management of patients with symptom magnification behaviors.

NIOSH once estimated that only 15% of low back pain (LBP) is diagnosed correctly. Even if that number were 30% or 50%, there would still be a substantial number of individuals with LBP who remain undiagnosed or improperly diagnosed. Most referrals from qualified physicians carry diagnoses such as lumbosacral sprain, lumbosacral sprain/strain, disc syndrome, LBP, and so on. This is expected since there is no universally accepted algorithm for evaluating persons complaining of LBP. Diagnostic procedures generally look at structure, not function. Therefore, precautions for treatment and restriction of activities of daily living (ADL) are usually determined in direct relationship to the patient or client's (p/c's) verbalization of their complaints. The more they complain, the greater are the limitations placed on their functional behavior. The best example of this is the individual complaining of LBP who has plenty of symptoms but absolutely no objective findings and who may be diagnosed as having a lumbosacral strain. It is disconcerting to treat such patients because their disability seems greater than it should be based on the objective findings. Twenty years ago, these patients would have been labeled "crocks," or "whiners." It was common belief that worker's compensation patients displayed these attributes more than "regular" patients. Therefore, our expectations of what they could accomplish were much lower than for regular patients. Our success was also diminished because our doubts about the validity of their complaints were apparent.

A particular patient from years ago comes to mind. This was an obese woman who was unemployed, on welfare, receiving Aid to Dependent Children, and seeing a psychiatrist three times per week for instruction on how to relax so she could sleep better. After performing an assessment which yielded absolutely no objective findings, I advised her to find employment, work a typical 8 to 10 hour day, and take care of her home and family. By the time she was ready to retire for the evening she couldn't do anything but sleep. You can imagine what she was like the next day when she arrived for her second treatment! She could hardly drag herself into the office, complaining of increased back pain and disability. I had put her in a position where she found it necessary to *prove* that she had a back problem—and prove it she did.

Who Is the Symptom Magnifier?

While there are many definitions of symptom magnification, I prefer a broad, simplified definition: the patient's response, or disability, is much greater than expected based on objective findings. Conceptually, almost everyone with LBP could be symptom magnifying to some degree. It is not a matter of if, but rather how much they are symptom magnifying. A symptom magnifier can be identified by performing a thorough history and physical.

Pain Scale Drawings

The history should include pain scale drawings which gives p/c's an opportunity to identify the nature and extent of their discomfort. It has been our experience that patients who have very few objective findings, but extensive symptoms, will complete the pain scale drawings in a predictable manner. We use a horizontal line, 10 centimeters long from left to right (see Figure 6.1). The extreme left side of the line represents a complete absence of pain. The extreme right side represents a maximum level of pain. The p/c is requested to indicate, with a vertical line intersecting the horizontal line, the pain at its absolute worst; at its absolute minimum; and where it is presently. Most symptom magnifiers (labeled SM in Figure 6.1) place all three marks to the far right on the pain scale. We know from our

Indicate on the pain scale below by making a line where your pain is at its least, worst; and where it is now:

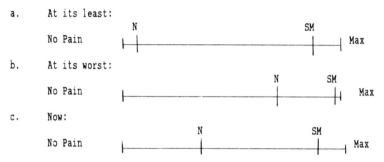

a.   At its least:

b.   At its worst:

c.   Now:

Figure 6.1 Pain scale drawing using a horizontal line, 10 centimeters long from left to right. The extreme left side of the line represents a complete absence of pain. The extreme right side of the line represents a maximum level of pain.

experience, personal and professional, that pain with a musculoskeletal origin should be close to, if not zero at rest or in some positions. The pattern of reporting pain by a p/c with minimal, if any, symptom magnification is labeled "N" on the pain scale in Figure 6.1. Other subjective pain drawings can also be used. For example, we use the outline of a body and ask p/c's to use the figure to indicate the type and position of their pain. A p/c who is symptom magnifying will either fill in the entire figure and draw marks with arrows directed into the figure or will place only one small dot in the figure (see Figure 6.2).

Waddell's Non-Organic Signs

It is important to observe the p/c's overt pain behavior such as facial grimacing, hand rubbing, or touching affected parts. Waddell's "Physical Signs in Non-Organic Low Back Pain," are also strong indicators of the magnitude of symptom magnification. (Gordon Waddell's "Nonorganic Physical Signs in Low-Back Pain," 1979 Volvo Award in Clinical Science can be found in the March/April 1980 issue of *Spine*.) In his study, Waddell states that if an individual is positive on three of the five broad categories of signs presented in his article, it is likely the patient's problem is predominantly of non-organic origin.

Tests of Maximum Voluntary Effort

There are a variety of tests for maximum voluntary effort (M.V.E.) to determine if the p/c is withholding effort, or symptom magnifying. A simple gross grip dynamometer can be used to look at the overall pat-

On the drawing below, use the *legend* to draw on the figure where your problem is located.

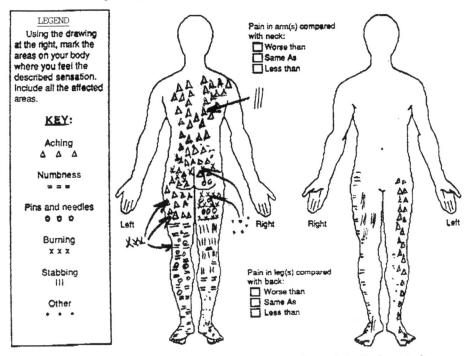

Figure 6.2 Pain drawing in which patients use an outline of the body to indicate the type and position of their pain.

tern of force the p/c produces in each of the five dynamometer positions. One would expect a bell-shaped curve. That is, the least amount of tension should be developed in positions 1 and 5. The greatest amount of tension should be developed in the mid-range. Our statistics show the mean *force* developed in position 3 utilizing a Jamar dynamometer by right-hand dominant males and females was 96 and 51 lbs. respectively.

Another test of M.V.E. is the p/c's ability to produce tension during a static lift on an arm/leg/chest dynamometer. Lifting with the back in lordosis, the p/c should be able to produce greater tension than lifting with the back in a kyphotic position. Our experience is that most women produce 22% more tension and men average 20% more tension with the lordic position.

Other objective measurements, such as the use of computerized dynamometers, can also help determine if a p/c is withholding effort. Inconsistent, or nonphysiological movement patterns in tension development can be documented easily with these instruments.

In utilizing functional tests such as standing, sitting, walking, lifting, pushing, pulling, carrying, and so on, the clinician should look for nonphysiological and inconsistent performances, especially in relationship to what has been discovered during the manual exam. These are just a few of the procedures that can be used to identify symptom magnifying behavior.

Secondary Financial Gain

Another factor in symptom magnification is the attorney. Suppose a blue-collar worker injures his back and visits health care practitioners and others who seem to question his sincerity. He's heard horror stories from friends and relatives about people who have had back problems and unfavorable outcomes. They suggest he consult with an attorney to determine whether he should take any legal action. The attorney *might* say something like this: "I know that you're a brave guy and that you don't think your problem is very significant. But I'd like to tell you I've seen many people with problems similar to yours who five years down the road have arthritis so bad they can't even get up out of a chair. How do you think you're going to provide for your family if that happens? How will you make your house and car payments? How will you provide for your children's education, clothing, and everything else? Now is the time for you to take action, not five years from now when it may be too late. Who do you think the doctor, the therapist, and the rehabilitation specialist represent, you? No! They are paid by your company. They represent your company! I'm the only person who represents *your* interest. I don't get paid unless you get paid." What do you think the chances are he might consider some type of legal action?

Patients who decide to institute some type of legal action are often told: "Be careful when you see those therapists. I know they mean well, but if you laugh at their jokes and act like you don't have a problem, they aren't going to believe your problem is serious. So you really should be on guard when you visit with these folks. If I were you, I would confine my activities. I wouldn't be going bowling or to shopping malls or other places where you might be seen." It would be nice to think that attorneys who say such things really don't understand what they are doing, but these are certainly instructions on how to become a depressed person. And by acting depressed, patients become depressed. Actions precede emotions. It is interesting that this is the profile we see in many of our p/c's, especially those involved in litigation.

There are a host of financial factors that may come into play as well. Many individuals have short-term disability policies that cover boat, car, and house payments, and possibly even a disability policy to supplement their income. These individuals may have realistic concerns regarding the long-term outcome of their injury from a financial perspective.

Other Contributing Factors

The medical system itself contributes to symptom magnification. The typical passive approach of prescribing pills and rest for as little as three or four days may actually create a chronic pain syndrome. Findings commensurate with age, such as degenerative disc disease and other "normal" findings, are misunderstood as being pathological. The more impressive the terminology applied to the problem sounds, the greater the severity as perceived by the p/c.

Managing Symptom Magnification

Helping the P/C Accept Help

Our approach to the management of symptom magnification is simple and forthright. It begins by legitimizing the p/c's feelings. We accept all complaints of pain as valid. Pain is a complex phenomenon and any perception of pain is real.

Perception is simply an internal representation of an external event. Things are as we perceive them to be. There is no way I can prove or disprove what individuals report regarding their experience of pain. So I choose to accept their perception. Take, for example, a p/c who sustained a back injury approximately one year ago. The patient has had every existing diagnostic study, some of them more than once, and has visited a host of medical professionals. No objective findings are evident and yet the patient is unable to work or engage in any recreational activities and is confined to basic self-care ADL.

Patients with this profile should be assisted in working through their situation until they understand that nothing more can be done medically. All pertinent diagnostic studies that can feasibly be performed have been performed and interpreted properly by competent physicians who are concerned about the p/c. Help the p/c to conclude there is no magic pill or surgery that will take care of the problem.

How to Explain Symptom Magnification

Having worked through the above, the p/c is now ready to have symptom magnification explained. We begin by discussing the various properties of pain such as the experience of, interpretation of, and reaction to pain. It might be helpful to use the following analogy. Suppose there are identical twins who decide to ride their mountain bikes straight up a mountain. One twin is an accomplished biker and a strong athlete. The other twin has led a sedentary life. As they proceed up the mountain, they will probably both feel a burning sensation in their thighs. This *experience* of discomfort is similar in both twins. The *interpretation* of pain by the athletic twin might be: "Great, my thighs are burning. I know I'm working hard." The nonathletic twin might interpret this pain as: "Something is wrong!" The athletic twin's *response* to the experience and interpretation of pain might be: "This is great. I'm going to work really hard and get a super workout." The nonathletic twin's reaction to the pain may be: "I think I should stop." At this point, patients may ask if the clinician believes they are lying or overreacting. The most helpful reply is to explain to the p/c that individuals respond differently to similar situations and may have different threshold tolerances to various stimuli. For example, some people can have a tooth drilled and filled without anesthetic. Others are white knuckled all the way. Emphasize that this is not meant to be judgmental; it's simply that people have different pain thresholds.

To demonstrate the process of symptom magnification using a noxious stimulus, we generally apply firm thumb pressure to the dorsum of the p/c's wrist or to the vastus medialis muscle. We then discuss the p/c's immediate experience. Their *interpretation* is often "Why is this person doing this?" Their *response* is usually to allow continued application of pressure without resistance. We ask the p/c how he or she would feel if the pressure were maintained for an extended period of time, for example, every minute of every day for the next four months. Would they experience more or less pain? The typical response is more pain. However, the accurate answer is less pain. If the p/c doubts this conclusion, we give the example of an amputation or some other traumatic experience the p/c may comprehend. Immediately following the incident, the pain associated with the injury is at its maximum. After a week or so, the pain has begun to decrease. At some point the pain is virtually absent.

Returning to the present problem and the scenario above, we ask what the patients' *interpretation* of this pain might be over a prolonged period of time. Typically, they report they would grow to intensely dislike the pain and their interpretation might be: "I want to relieve myself of this pain. I would pull your hand off of my wrist or knee." They might even wish to retaliate. By this time patients have admitted there is no magic pill or surgery that can take care of their problem; they understand the process of symptom magnification and that they may be engaging in that process, at least to some extent.

Identification of Disincentives to Recovery

The next question to ask patients is whether they would really like to get better. This almost invariably causes a strong reaction. Most often the reply is: "Of course, I want to get better. Why do you think I've gone to all those doctors?" Another question to ask is what they stand to lose if they get better. What are the benefits of staying disabled? Perhaps by remaining disabled they have more freedom to determine their daily schedule. They may receive sympathy from friends and relatives. They may obtain a disability rating which will enable them to receive an income without working. They may also have reprieve from household chores. There may be other factors which are more sensitive such as engaging in substance abuse. They may have an abusive spouse who is not abusive as long as they are disabled. It is important for the p/c to recognize these possibilities. We believe admitting that there are things to lose if they get better is the first step to identifying those factors so we can work with the p/c to eliminate those disincentives. In my experience, this has been the most difficult area for p/c's to face. At times, it takes them several days to come up with factors that may be an impediment to their improvement. Fostering a nonjudgmental environment and encouraging p/c's to talk about the issues that affect their situation will facilitate responsiveness. There are times when this process will yield "go for help" signs. These include verbalization regarding suicide, physical abuse toward another, substance abuse, sexual problems, and others that may be outside a clinician's area of expertise.

Helping the P/C's Take Responsibility for Their Health

At this point, we explain to p/c's what are, apparently, their obvious choices and responsibilities. Their choice may be to hurt and be nonfunctional which is usually what brought them to the office, or to hurt and be functional. I know a person who had a back problem for more than 20 years. Eleven years ago after a boating mishap he had a complete foot drop on the left which resulted in laminectomies at two levels. He experienced complications after surgery that slowed recovery. He was categorized as a failed back surgery. He experienced almost continual LBP which was exacerbated by almost any physical activity. It occurred to him that if he was going to hurt anyway, maybe he'd be better off hurting and doing something that he enjoyed such as bike riding or cross-country skiing. This was the beginning of his taking control of his situation. He has done well ever since with regard to his ADL though he still experiences LBP. This may be an oversimplification, but if p/c's have plenty of symptoms and no signs, what is the risk of their being active? They hurt anyway, so if they are active and hurt, they are certainly better off. And, if the activity causes the pathology to extend itself, it's quite possible that might even be beneficial because the pathology could then be identified. It's also important to explain to p/c's the difference between hurt and harm with regard to their problem. If they have been nonfunctional for quite some time, it's likely their flexibility, strength, and endurance are at less than an optimal level. Therefore, when they begin a work hardening program, it's likely they will become sore and this will hurt. Consider the person who lays off playing softball all winter and when spring arrives, starts practicing again. Throwing the ball may make the arm sore and that will hurt. But it doesn't cause any harm. The soreness will go away after a period of time.

We then explain to the p/c two main categories of factors that are involved in their situation—factors they can control and factors they can't control. The choice they have is to continue to complain about things they cannot control, which has no positive outcome, or to choose to change the things they are able to change. We are trying to create an awareness that everything p/c's do is because of a choice they make. The choices they can make will determine the quality of the rest of their life. So if their choice is to participate in a work hardening or other treatment program, we require they accept responsibility for the program including showing up at the appointed time, being consistent and persistent with their treatments, giving a good effort, and establishing other criterion for their participation in the program.

Patients are then given a brochure explaining the work hardening program. It includes a definition of work hardening, along with the procedures in which they will be involved to accomplish the established goals. Their responsibilities are outlined and include when and where the program takes place, the importance of being on time, what to wear, and what results they can expect. The p/c is then required to sign a contract, similar to the one in Figure 6.3, to more formally establish a desire to participate in the program. The p/c is informed that noncompliance with the agreement is a reason for discharge from the program (prior agreement by the referral source is always obtained).

Motivation

We try to accomplish all of the above during the first work hardening session. Throughout the work hardening regime, we do our utmost to motivate and inspire the p/c. We try to make the experience enjoyable, to help p/c's realize the possibilities that exist through making choices and their responsibility to determine what choices they make. For example, we might say during one of the early visits: "Right now, I know there is no place on earth that you would rather be than right here." Of course, they look at us like we're crazy and say: "Oh yeah. Well, I'd rather be in Alaska." Our response might be: "Why don't you go?" This is met with excuses such as: "I don't have enough money;" I can't take the time off;" "Worker's Com-

---

RETURN TO WORK
PROCESS "CONTRACT"

I, _____ , have had the Return to Work Process explained to me in detail. I have also received my "Work Hardening and You" brochure.

Furthermore, I will put forth an honest effort. I understand that the intent of the program is not designed to eliminate my pain, but to increase my ability to perform work-related activities.

It has been explained to me that the program will start promptly at 8:00 a.m. unless it has been approved beforehand to arrive late. There will be a lunch break at 12:00 noon and the program will resume at 1:00 p.m. sharp. My program will end each day as designated by a professional staff person. If I am late I will call to speak to a professional staff member and will continue to call until I reach that person.

Signed _____

Witness _____

Date _____

Figure 6.3 Return to work process "contract."

pensation will not pay;" and many others. Realizing there are solutions to those excuses, at some point they admit: "Well, maybe I'd rather stay here in this city than go to Alaska." Again, we may respond: "Why don't you just go home?" The response may be: "Well, they won't pay for my worker's compensation if I go home."

We reply, "So you would rather be here and get paid than go home and not get paid." I'm sure you see our intention. Through a series of questions, we'll assist p/c's to realize that indeed it is their choice to be here. Nobody is putting a gun to their head and it is only by their choice that they actually show up for treatment. Now, we present another choice. How much do they choose to get out of the treatment regime? They can choose to come in and waste their time and get nothing out of it, or they can choose to work hard and improve. Patients begin to realize that we are going to be honest with them and everyone involved with their case. We don't hide any facts or have any secret communications between ourselves and others involved with their case. We are consistent in our approach and are also direct with them regarding these factors. We may explain what we mean by victim mentality and tell them they have a choice—to either maintain their attitude as a victim or to extinguish the victim mentality. Again, it is their choice.

It helps to have motivational posters in your office such as a Nike "Just Do It" poster. There are many different posters that are commercially available. The most important aspect of the poster is the motto and not the art value of the poster. Some posters have mottos such as: "If it is to be, it's up to me;" "I can if I think I can;" "Only those who risk going too far can actually determine how far they can go;" and "Real winners are ordinary people with extraordinary determination." We generally ask p/c's what the mottos on the motivational posters mean to them. For example, if the poster states "Just Do It" we might ask: "What does this mean to you?" A typical response is: "Nothin'." If this is the case, we ask them to try to come up with something they could tell us with regard to their own lives in relation to the motto on the poster. No matter how reluctant some p/c's are, after a period of time they get the idea and begin to exert some control over their lives by establishing goals and plans to achieve them. This does not happen overnight and it doesn't happen to every p/c, but it does happen to a good portion of them.

This has been a description of how we manage the patient and manage symptom magnification. All of this may seem a bit elementary; however, it has been our experience that if insufficient attention is paid to these details, the program will not be as successful as it could be. It has also been our experience that most clinicians give lip service to understanding these principles, but few put them into action.

Work Hardening

Historical Perspectives

The late 1970s and early 1980s brought a realization that traditional therapies for work-related injuries were not sufficient to restore patients to their preinjury status with little risk of reinjury to themselves or compromising the safety of others. There was also a suspicion by third-party payors and employers that many injured employees were malingerers. These factors combined to create the need for work hardening. Employers and third-party payors liked the term and concept of work hardening. It represented a departure from traditional approaches to back problems. It meant no more hot packs and massage, no more pills and rest. Somehow the term work hardening implied the outcome would be the p/c returning to gainful employment. This concept slowly gained popularity. By the late 1980s and early 1990s, nearly everyone was providing work hardening programs. This has caused considerable confusion among third-party payors and employers paying for these procedures. What is meant by work hardening and how is its effectiveness determined?

Ultimately, third-party payors will determine the "quality" of care by evaluating the total cost to resolve the case of an injured employee. Like it or not, that's probably a reasonable way to determine a program's effectiveness. After all, it is the intent of the program to assist in the process of case resolution.

The Program Overview

Our program can be defined as a series of goal-directed supervised activities, designed to improve the functional performance of participants. The program includes a physical reconditioning component to improve the p/c's flexibility, strength, and endurance; an educational segment including instruction in proper body mechanics, stress management, nutritional habits, and so on; and work simulation which duplicates the p/c's specific job tasks.

Determination of Work Hardening Intensity and Progression

The intensity of the work hardening program depends on p/c's level of symptom magnification. If p/c's are engaging in minimal symptom magnification, they are started closer to physiological levels of exercise intensity than those engaging in maximum symptom magnification. Those engaging in maximum symptom magnification begin the program at a level low enough to assure their success and not extend their injury or cause them harm. For example, a p/c with no objective findings but considerable complaints might begin on a gentle stretching program not involving the back but including stretching of the gastroc soleus, upper extremity, head, and neck. The total stretching program might last only four or five minutes. The strengthening program might involve exercise that does not directly affect the back such as the chest press, rowing machine, and LAT pull-downs. Three or four of these machines may be utilized during the first session. The resistance on these machines would generally be 10 to 15 pounds or less and one set performed with only five or six repetitions. The aerobic phase might utilize a treadmill set at a speed of 1.2 miles per hour. The duration of exercise on the treadmill might be less than 5 minutes. Obviously, p/c's who don't have any objective findings would have to work to hurt themselves on such a regime. These p/c's are usually amazed at how little work they actually performed. Many times they comment, "Is that all?" They may even ask if they can perform more. Occasionally p/c's may complain of pain caused by these exercises. If we are absolutely sure that the nature of the exercises was such that they could not extend or create an injury, we remind them that the program is not designed to address pain. They are again, in a friendly nonjudgmental fashion, informed of the choices they have regarding their condition. The first reconditioning session may only last 30 minutes. Initially, we feel it is important to put p/c's into a position where they can't help but succeed. *They are slowly progressed during every single treatment.* We may increase the reps, sets, resistance, and machines used in the weight training program. Gradually, we increase the time spent stretching and increase the duration and intensity of the strengthening and aerobic exercises. Over a short period of time, p/c's begin to demonstrate improvement in their ability to tolerate exercise. By the end of the first week, the reconditioning session usually lasts 1 hour. By the end of the second week, the reconditioning session may be 2 hours. At this point, the duration is held constant and the intensity is increased each subsequent session. Patients begin to look and feel better about themselves and start to exhibit control over their situation.

In several weeks, they are performing a stretching program that lasts approximately 30 minutes and are performing two or three sets of 10 to 15 repetitions on each of our machines which generally takes them approximately an hour to perform. Within several weeks the intensity of the aerobic phase increases so the p/c's target heart rate is maintained for 45 minutes to 1 hour.

Patients are progressed until their performance is commensurate with the physical demand characteristics of the job category (or specific job) for which they are training. Consideration is given to a "margin of safety" as suggested by NIOSH (that is, regarding worksite lifting requirements, an occasional lift [meaning up to 20 minutes of every hour] should not exceed 50% of maximum lifting capacity; a frequent lift [20 to 40 minutes of every hour] should not exceed 25% of maximum lifting capacity; continuous lifting [more than 40 minutes of every hour] should not exceed 10% of maximum lifting capacity).

Education

Every day p/c's receive educational information including instruction in proper body mechanics, responsibility for their own well-being, basic anatomy, and other subjects. The purpose is to present concepts from a wide variety of sources that support the process of managing symptom magnification as previously described. These sources could include videotapes of TV programs related to back care or general health. They may include inspirational tapes (Zig Ziglar, Wayne Dyer, Dennis Wheatly, and others) that can be obtained through Nightingale-Conant Corporation, 7300 North Lehigh Avenue, Chicago, IL 60648. These occupy 30 to 60 minutes per day and are combined whenever possible with other activities.

Work Simulation

The work simulation program is designed to simulate those forces required by the physical characteristics of the p/c's job. This is achieved through the use of basic work stations and cooperation with the

---

NAME _____

DATE _____

JOB DESCRIPTION _____

_____

_____

_____

DIAGRAM OF ACTIVITIES (SKETCH)

EQUIPMENT UTILIZED _____

\+   REPS. _____   WEIGHTS _____

TIME LIMIT _____

COMPLAINTS _____

COMMENTS _____

_____

_____

Figure 6.4 Work simulation log used to record the patient's activity during the work simulation phase of the work hardening program.

employer in obtaining tools or devices that the employee uses on the job. In order to approximate the physical demands, it may be necessary to perform a job site analysis. The physical characteristics include the forces required to push/pull, lift, and so on, and the frequency and duration of application of those forces. At the very least, a "walk-through" job site analysis should be

---

NAME _____

DATE _____

JOB DESCRIPTION _____

_____

_____

_____

DIAGRAM OF ACTIVITIES (SKETCH)

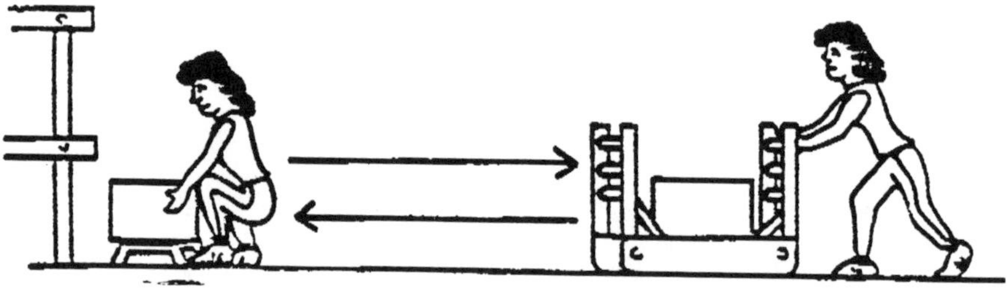

EQUIPMENT UTILIZED _____

+   REPS. _____   WEIGHTS _____

TIME LIMIT _____

COMPLAINTS _____

COMMENTS _____

_____

_____

Figure 6.5 Work simulation log used to record the patient's activity during the work simulation phase of the work hardening program.

done to approximate the various components of work-related activities. The work simulation can be designed by reading a thorough job description. While these last two methods are least desirable, occasionally employers are unwilling to pay for a thorough job site analysis. As the Americans with Disabilities Act of 1990 takes effect with regard to employment, employers will be more willing to pay for a thorough job site analysis. The most effective method to obtain approval to perform a job site analysis is to explain to the payor and employer that before you can determine when a p/c can return to work, you must know what physical demands must be met. A recommended guideline for charging for this service is to charge what you would bill if you

NAME _____

DATE _____

JOB DESCRIPTION _____
_____
_____
_____

DIAGRAM OF ACTIVITIES (SKETCH)

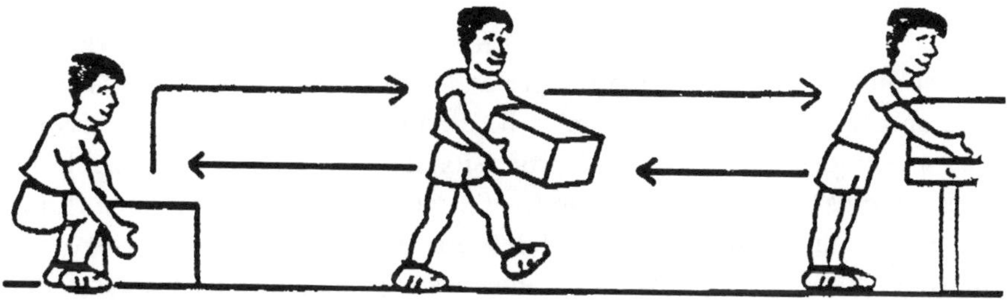

EQUIPMENT UTILIZED _____

+   REPS. _____   WEIGHTS _____

TIME LIMIT _____

COMPLAINTS _____

COMMENTS _____
_____
_____

Figure 6.6 Work simulation log used to record the patient's activity during the work simulation phase of the work hardening program.

were seeing the p/c in your clinic for that same period of time. Progression with the work simulation component of the work hardening program follows the same philosophy as the reconditioning component. The duration of the first session is about 2 hours, including the reconditioning component. By the end of the second week, the duration is a full day (less two 15 minute breaks and lunch). The intensity is then increased until the p/c is able to perform at the physical level required by the job using the criterion previously mentioned. Figures 6.4, 6.5, and 6.6 are used to record the p/c's activity during the work simulation phase of the work hardening program. The actual recording is performed by the program supervisor. This makes it easier for one "Work Capacity Specialist" to supervise up to five p/c's at a time. Within a few weeks, the employee is working a full 8-hour day (2 hours of reconditioning and 6 hours of work simulation) at our clinic. Generally, this is at a greater intensity than the p/c would actually perform at work. This seems to provide motivation for the individual to return to work. Our approach is one of considerable flexibility; whether or not a p/c participates in both the physical conditioning and work simulation components, and for how long, is determined on an individual basis. Our goal is to help resolve each case as efficiently as possible.

Conclusion

There is no magic in these procedures, but they work. The greatest difficulty in managing the p/c and symptom magnification is reluctance on the part of the clinician to be direct with the p/c and discuss the areas mentioned above. Medical professionals seem to feel responsible for making the patient better. We tend to assume responsibility for those things that are only under the p/c's control. It seems we want to be in control of the situation and be the caregiver, thus encouraging the p/c to be the caretaker. This creates dependency on the medical system in general and on our treatment program and ourselves in particular. Instead, we need to empower p/c's to take responsibility for their own well-being. We believe the management program described above provides this empowerment.

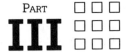

Functional
Considerations

Part III, Functional Considerations, presents successful LBP re-habilitation in light of specific functional impairments and their objective measurements. The distinction between disability claims and physical impairments is becoming increasingly recognized by a more sophisticated health care industry. While it is often unclear why specific impairments persist, the role of muscular endurance in perpetuating impairments is gaining greater clinical recognition. Electromyographic measures of fatigue offer both a physiologic view of the process and a more specific anatomical identification of the muscles involved. The consequences of these physiologic changes, detailed in chapter 7, The Role of Muscle Fatigue in Low Back Pain, are often measured in functional capacities examinations. While research validation of functional capacities examinations is eagerly awaited by clinicians, there is a substantive empirical base behind their performance. Many functional capacities examination measurements are well standardized and are widely accepted by insurance carriers. While clinical approaches to rehabilitation are varied, it is interesting to note the trend in industrial medicine toward standardized specific functional capacities examination procedures, such as those presented in chapter 8, Advancements in Functional Capacity Evaluation.

To a great extent, an accurate measurement of impairment is predicated on patients performing each task near their maximum capabilities. Many methods to validate the patient's effort have been documented over the last ten years. One of the most promising pieces of equipment toward this end is the trunk dynamometer. Much as isokinetic testing advanced functional examination of upper and lower extremity strength in the 1970s, the late 1980s and early 1990s are witnessing a similar advancement with the trunk. To avoid pitfalls in data interpretation, the clinician needs to be aware of engineering limitations with trunk dynamometers which are presented in chapter 9, Objective Quantification of Trunk Performance. By examining these specific engineering concepts and integrating these concepts into a clinical picture, the clinician can provide a far more accurate view of the patient's function when combined with other clinical forms of examination. In time, trunk dynamometers will assist in validating claims of successful treatment and already have proven themselves valuable in guiding rehabilitation programs through objective feedback. Many examples of objective feedback are given in chapter 10, Case Reports: Use of Trunk Dynamometers in the Management of Patients with Spinal Disorders.

7

□□□
□□□
□□□

The Role of Muscle Fatigue in Low Back Pain

Serge H. Roy

In a recent workshop comprised of internationally recognized researchers in the field of low back pain (LBP), guidelines for future research in LBP were discussed.[1] It is relevant to the topic of this chapter that the workshop placed far greater emphasis on the role of muscles in LBP than did a similar workshop convened eight years earlier.[2] New information from improved methods of assessing muscle function has resulted in a renewed interest in assessing the muscular component of back pain. With this renewed interest comes the prospect that we may be closer to identifying the relationship between muscle dysfunction and low back pain.

This chapter focuses on the role of muscle fatigue in LBP. Muscle fatigue can severely compromise the dual function of back muscles to (1) maintain the stability of the vertebral column and (2) control spinal movement. Despite its importance as a mechanism that affects function, muscle fatigue as a process is poorly understood. Muscle fatigue is a complex process that lacks a universal definition. Numerous mechanisms involving multiple sites have been associated with fatigue. In spite of the ability to distinguish different sites or mechanisms of fatigue, nonspecific terminology is often used to describe fatigue.

Measurement of fatigue in research and clinical studies has been relegated primarily to limb musculature rather than to paraspinal muscles. Only recently have fatigue measurement techniques been applied to low back musculature. The current commercial proliferation of isometric and isodynamic dynamometers in the clinical and research environments attests to the need for more objective measurement of muscle function. Other objective techniques to assess fatigue rely on the use of surface electromyography (EMG).

Surface EMG has evolved in the laboratory to the point where it can be considered a viable adjunct to more conventional clinical procedures for assessing muscle dysfunction. Further elaboration on these techniques is presented later in this chapter where spectral analysis of EMG signals detected from lumbar electrode arrays is described.

The emergence of industrial medicine has provided an impetus toward more sophisticated instrumentation to assess muscle impairment. The failure of previous conventional approaches to assess and treat work-related back injuries has resulted in the current trend toward work hardening. This approach emphasizes the physical demands of the work environment as they impact the functional capability of the musculoskeletal system. Work-related tasks are studied in terms of their mechanical demands on the passive and active components of the spine. Because almost every task is time dependent, the endurance capacity of the musculature is a key component to the system. Muscle performance is therefore considered not only in terms of the immediate capability of a muscle to generate force but also in terms of how well a muscle can sustain the required force during repeated activation (that is, while doing work). If the muscle can no longer maintain the tension demanded by the task, injury to the muscle and other structures may ensue. Consider the value to a physical therapist or other clinician in being able to monitor the development of fatigue in individual muscle groups during work or while replicating a key component of that work. Furthermore, identifying which muscles are dysfunctional and to what degree can provide the basis for a tailored exercise program to restore the level of function needed for a particular task. The extent to which we can currently accomplish this objective will be examined in this chapter.

Defining Fatigue

Fatigue is a term that has been defined in many ways, usually depending on how one chooses to measure it. The definition of fatigue should therefore be considered operational; that is, it is intimately related to the process being monitored. Classically, fatigue has been described in terms of the ability of a muscle to sustain a particular level of force output. In this instance, one would monitor muscle tension either via an *in vitro* preparation or via the torque or some other convenient measure of mechanical output from the muscle. Fatigue would therefore be measured in units of time that transpired until the target force level or mechanical output could no longer be sustained. Similarly, if a task were being repeated until the individual could no longer produce another repetition, then fatigue would be measured in units of the number of repetitions. There are numerous other examples from the clinical environment. A very different, but equally acceptable approach is to define fatigue as a continuous, time-dependent process. Fatigue in this instance is continually occurring from the moment a contraction begins. This definition is more consistent with how an engineer defines fatigue. A good example of this approach is described by Basmajian and De Luca who use the analogy of measuring fatigue in the steel girders of a bridge to describe muscle fatigue.[3] Fatigue in the steel girders occurs continuously. Microscopic conformational changes take place in the molecular bonds of the steel that gradually weaken the bridge's structure over time even though one cannot observe a change in the bridge's ability to remain standing. These authors make the point that according to the classical approach, the bridge would have to collapse before "fatigue" was present. From a purely practical point of view, it is more useful for the engineer to monitor changes in the steel girders that precede the mechanical failure of the system than to monitor the bridge as it collapses. This analogy can be applied to describing fatigue in a muscle. Time-dependent processes such as the metabolic and electrophysiological changes that occur during a sustained contraction may be monitored and defined as fatigue parameters because they are precursors to eventual mechanical failure of the muscle.

Measurements of muscle force or other related parameters of mechanical output such as torque can be monitored in a way that is consistent with the definition of fatigue as a continuous process. An example of this is to serially monitor the decrement in the maximal force generating capacity of a muscle. Each of the two operational definitions of fatigue have advantages and disadvantages that will dictate which is more appropriate for a particular objective. The most obvious advantage of the time-dependent measure of fatigue is that the subject need not sustain a task until the point of mechanical failure (exhaustion) of the muscle. This advantage may be particularly desirable in evaluating patient populations because it limits the stress on an already compromised musculoskeletal system. Secondly, in those instances in which the fatigue parameter is not defined in terms of the force output of the muscle, the subject's performance is less likely to be influenced by psychological factors or pain inhibition. Models of fatigue that rely on a singular event such as mechanical failure do have one advantage: they can be measured with minimal instrumentation. This is one reason why this approach has been common in clinical practice. This advantage is less persuasive now that simplified new techniques and instrumentation are available.

The definition of fatigue in this discussion has been limited to processes occurring at the muscular level. This approach has been referred to as *peripheral muscle fatigue* or *localized muscle fatigue*.[4] These terms emphasize that events are limited to mechanisms peripheral to the neuromuscular junction, for example, at the sarcolemma or intracellularly. All other processes taking place in the central nervous system, including psychogenic

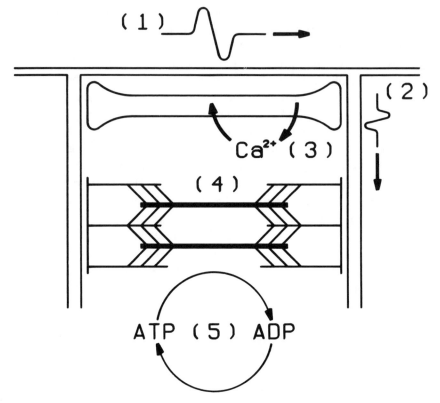

Figure 7.1 Diagram illustrating the primary sites of fatigue localized to the muscle. These sites are indicated in the diagram as the (1) muscle membrane; (2) T-tubule; (3) sarcoplasmic reticulum; (4) actin-myosin coupling; and (5) muscle energetics.

components are categorized as *central fatigue* and are not emphasized in this discussion. Clinicians and researchers have difficulty measuring central fatigue. Although they may try to limit its effect on peripheral mechanisms of fatigue, they cannot completely eliminate it except in the extreme case of an *in vitro* study.

Peripheral sites of failure in the muscular system can be further divided into contractile, metabolic, or electrophysiological fatigue. Figure 7.1 depicts the location of these sites in a simplified form. Contractile failure is most likely to occur during excitation contraction coupling (sites 2 and 3) or during the formation of actin-myosin complex (site 4). Metabolic failure can occur at each of the sites depicted in Figure 7.1 either as a result of insufficient ATP production or as a result of inhibiting key enzymes or contractile processes when metabolites such as H^+, K^+, or P_i accumulate within the muscle. Cardiovascular fitness, although more of a systemic process, influences peripheral metabolic processes necessary for the production of ATP and impacts the elimination of metabolites. Cardiovascular fitness and LBP will be discussed in greater detail later in this chapter.

Electrophysiological failure is primarily relegated to site 1 in Figure 7.1 and can occur through a reduced excitability of the sarcolemma, resulting in a slowing or change in the length of the depolarized zone, which will be recorded as changes in the EMG signal shape (commonly referred to as the *signal waveform*). For a more detailed explanation of these processes refer to any of several excellent reviews published recently[5,6] or to textbooks of muscle physiology.[7,8]

Anatomical and Physiological Characteristics of Lumbar Muscles

Most scientific reports concerning skeletal muscles are based on limb muscles rather than spinal musculature. Information derived from these studies can be extrapolated to back muscles to identify the role of fatigue in LBP. Anatomical properties of back muscles are highly specialized to provide high levels of force that can be sustained over long periods of time for the purpose of maintaining posture or producing motion. The amount of force required to maintain postural stability against gravity, even when relatively moderate loads are carried, can be quite high. For example, it is estimated that the erector spinae must generate 800 N of force during lifting of a 10 kg load at arm's length.[9] Forces of this magnitude are provided structurally by large muscle masses with many parallel fibers. Back extensor muscles are larger in total mass than any other muscles in the body. Fibers typically span several joints and often function in an eccentric mode which further increases their tension-producing capacity. Most back extensor muscles overlap one another in a sequential arrangement and share common insertions to the lumbodorsal fascia. The lumbodorsal fascia is a thick tendonous band that can withstand tensile forces on the same order of magnitude as the muscle. These anatomical features may help disperse the high levels of force so they are not isolated to a few fibers.[10] This advantage, however, is dependent on a highly developed motor control system to coordinate the activation of many different muscle groups. In fact, the second anatomical feature of back muscles is that they contain a tremendous variety and number of separate muscle groups. There is evidence that this variety allows for a "rotation" effect whereby muscles can alternate in sustaining force to limit the development of fatigue in any one muscle. Rotation effects have been studied and identified in limb muscles, but understanding of this behavior is limited at best. One disadvantage of such complexity is that any impairment in the ability to provide control might lead to injury or a delay in recovery. One of the most difficult questions facing researchers studying the role of back muscles in LBP is whether muscle dysfunction is a problem of muscle control or a result of peripheral adaptation to injury and change in activity.

Most histochemical information from paravertebral muscle indicates that paraspinal muscles are well adapted to resist fatigue. Some caution is needed when appraising this information because many studies suffer from poor descriptions of their subject material and/or small numbers of subjects encompassing a wide range of ages. The site of biopsy sampling is often imprecise as well. For example, Sulemana et al. sampled 11 patients between the ages of 22 and 73 years using autopsy material from erector spinae muscle in which the site of sampling was not specified.[11] The mean ratio of Type I to Type II fibers was 1.76 and the mean cross-sectional area of Type I to Type II was 1.17. Autopsy studies from 21 adult male subjects (aged 22 to 46 years) combined with biopsy data from 12 males and 5 female subjects (aged between 28 to 50 years) reported a significantly greater proportion of Type I compared to Type II fibers in the thoracic level and nearly equal proportions in the lumbar area or when comparing superficial with deep layers of paraspinal muscles.[12] Other results from this study confirmed that Type I fibers are larger than Type II fibers in lumbar paraspinal muscles but not thoracic. These data suggest that a functional difference may exist between thoracic and lumbar paraspinals. More importantly, paraspinal muscles appear to have a physiological capability of resisting fatigue. As the summary of histological results reported for paraspinal muscles shows (see Table 7.1), back muscles have a high proportion of Type I muscle fibers with relatively large cross-sectional areas. These properties attest to the postural function of paraspinal muscles which must combine fatigue resistance with high levels of tension. Whether or not individuals with LBP have a higher proportion of paraspinal muscles with more easily fatigable Type II fibers than Type I fibers is still speculative. Biopsy data has been limited to spinal disc surgery patients and is often complicated by conflicting data regarding muscle fiber type composition as well as morphology.[12-15] Evidence for selective atrophy of muscle fiber types in LBP patients is consistent with reports in animals[16] and humans[17] that immobilization or disuse results in progressive atrophy of muscle fibers and modification of enzyme structure, limiting oxidative capacity. Preferential Type II atrophy may result when disuse is caused by pain or arthropathy, because pain may inhibit the rapid and more forceful contraction of Type II muscle fibers while still allowing the slower and less forceful contraction of Type I fibers.[10] Further histochemical studies are needed to verify whether congenital and adaptive features of paraspinal muscle fiber type are related to back injury.

Table 7.1 Reported Fiber Type Distribution and Mean Size of Muscle Fibers in Lumbar Paraspinal Muscles

Reference	N	Subjects	Muscle	Type I (%)	Mean Size (μm) Type I	Type II
Sirca et al.[12]	21*	Normal	Longissimus T9			
			superficial	74	53	53
			deep	73	50	47
			Multifidus L3			
			superficial	57	58	48
			deep	63	55	42
	17†	LBP	Multifidus L3			
			superficial	56	45	35
			deep	63	50	40
Bagnall et al.[13] and Ford et al.[14]	18†	LBP	Multifidus			
			superficial	53	62	37
			deep	49	59	41
Fidler et al.[15]	20†	LBP and normal	Multifidus	67		

*Autopsy data

†Biopsy data

Muscle Injury and Fatigue

Understanding of acute lumbosacral strain is hindered by the fact that the source of pain and initial site of injury are unknown. In contrast to the large amount of basic and clinical knowledge regarding injury to bone and ligaments, surprisingly little scientific information is available concerning injury to skeletal muscle. Back muscle tissue is subject to direct and indirect injury that can, at least in theory, be aggravated by muscle fatigue. Muscle fatigue can decrease the muscular support to the spine and result in increased mechanical stress to its functional components.[18] External loads are transmitted more readily to the soft tissue of the spine when the paraspinal musculature loses its ability to generate tension as a result of fatigue. Pain, joint effusion, anxiety, and lack of motivation can also result in a decrement of muscle force, which can also lead to an increased likelihood of injury. Reports of increased incidence of LBP in workers exposed to whole-body vibration[19] or repeated heavy manual tasks[20] support the theory that fatigue is associated with injury. Studies targeted at the work environment have demonstrated that muscle fatigue can impair motor coordination and control.[20] Muscle and connective tissue adapt rapidly to modified tension levels, which can result in a fixed structural disposition to injury. Among the relatively few studies that have investigated the process of indirect muscle injury, some research findings suggest that paraspinal muscles are predisposed to this type of injury.[10] Indirect muscle injury is synonymous with muscle strain and is defined as indirect injury to the myotendinous or osseotendinous junction caused by excessive tension, stretching, or a combination of both.

Clinical and experimental studies of strain injuries in extremity muscles have indicated that injury usually occurs as a response to excessive load or stretch and is most common during eccentric (muscle lengthening) contractions in muscles that span two or more joints.[21] Paraspinal muscles usually cross two or more vertebral levels and are usually preloaded eccentrically during lifting. Several anatomical features of motor units may also contribute to the high incidence of low back pain.[10] A concentration of motor units may produce strong localized forces which could result in strains and tissue damage.[22] Secondly, if each muscle fiber is connected to a common tendon rather than an individual tendon segment, the resulting strain would be more severe since it would be proportional to the sum total of muscles activated. Because muscle fibers are often arranged serially, there is an increased likelihood of strain occurring if an activated fiber were in series with an inactive fiber. This possibility would be determined by the recruitment order and anatomical arrangement of the muscle units.[23]

Strengthening, conditioning, "warming-up," and stretching of muscles is popularly believed to reduce the likelihood of muscle injury.[24,25] Epidemiological studies that have considered these muscular factors are inconclusive in verifying whether this belief is valid.[26] A few experimental studies have determined that muscle activation may protect muscle and limit strain injury by limiting the transference of loads to soft tissue.[10,26] The effect of preconditioning or warm-up has also been studied, and it was demonstrated that the force to rupture was increased in preconditioned rabbit muscles (via maximum isometric contraction) when compared to a control group.[27]

Back Muscle Fatigue and LBP

The role of muscle fatigue in the development and treatment of LBP has been of interest for at least the past two decades and still remains an enigma. Previous studies of fatigue in paraspinal muscles can be divided into mechanical studies of fatigue (i.e., endurance, failure to maintain a posture, sustaining a static torque or pace of work) or physiological studies of fatigue (e.g., biochemical and electromyographical). The majority of studies reported have been mechanical. Among the physiological studies, only EMG has been studied clinically. Currently, no biochemical studies specific to the back have been done. A few studies have compared EMG measures of fatigue with mechanical correlates. With the recent development of magnetic resonance spectroscopy for measuring high energy phosphate metabolites *in vivo* it may be possible to measure biochemical events noninvasively in back muscles during exercise.[28]

The simplest mechanical tests of back endurance have included maintaining a posture[29-32] and repeating an activity.[33-35] Biering-Sorensen popularized a static postural endurance test requiring subjects to maintain the prone, unsupported trunk in extension for as long as possible.[31] This test, described as "the couch method" was first introduced by Hansen.[36] Nicolaisen and Jorgensen used a similar test and found that patients with LBP had significantly shorter endurance times than controls.[37] Interestingly, isometric back strength did not differ between the two groups. They postulated that this result was an indication that the composition of back muscles in the patients was dominated by a greater proportion of easily fatigable Type II fibers. Other studies by these researchers found that back muscles in normal individuals have a relatively longer endurance capacity than other muscle groups of the body.[32] They attributed this difference to fiber composition of the muscle (primarily Type I) and increased blood perfusion, although this was not verified. In this study it was reported that subjects with prior occurrences of LBP were less endurant than but of similar strength to normal subjects. Nicolaisen and Jorgensen found similar results in another static endurance test in which the subject was required to maintain an isometric extension at 60% of maximum voluntary contraction (MVC) for as long as possible.[37] In a more recent work, this same group of researchers compared two methods for determining trunk extensor endurance.[38] Method I was the prone-lying trunk extension technique applied by Beiring-Sorensen[31] and Method II was "the pulling test" introduced by Jorgensen[39] in which the standing subject exerted a 60% MVC horizontal pull on a strain-gauge dynamometer. The time until complete exhaustion in either method was determined. Method I also had a 4-minute time constraint. The methods were applied to healthy male (n = 53) and female (n = 23) postal workers and 10 male students. The results demonstrated that Method II was preferable to Method I in terms of having less variability and a more normal distribution in the results, less dependence on physique, and shorter endurance times. The authors recommended Method II as an inexpensive and effective means of measuring trunk extensor endurance.

Triaxial dynamometers have also been used to study endurance. These devices measure the torque, velocity, and position of the trunk simultaneously in three planes. Constant loads can also be preset in each plane of movement to monitor torque, velocity, and displacement as the subject tries to overcome the preset load of the device. Nordin and associates measured torque, angular positions, and angular velocities while their subjects were tested isoinertially in an upright posture using a B-200 Isostation Dynamometer (Isotechnologies, Inc., Hillsborough, NC).[29,35] Endurance was measured by requiring subjects to move repeatedly in flexion and extension until fatigue developed. They reported that the ranges of movement were significantly affected by fatigue. During flexion and extension tests there were increased secondary movements in the coronal and transverse planes as the muscles fatigued. The researchers interpreted these results as evidence that fatigue leads to impairment of control and coordination. It was found that motion in the primary (sagittal) plane diminished with the onset of fatigue. These results demonstrated the inability of the neuromuscular system to accurately reproduce movements during fatigue. Impairment of motor control was also observed by a reduction of maximal and average velocities in the primary plane with a concomitant increase of velocities in the secondary (coronal) plane. It was argued in this study that the deleterious effects to the neuromuscular system associated with fatigue might predispose individuals to back injury. Few studies have investigated limited control or abnormal coupling in patients with low back pain.[40-42] Preliminary findings indicate that secondary axes torques are significantly lower for LBP patients compared to normal controls. This finding supports the belief that LBP results in a "guarding" phenomenon. Secondary axes information from tests of this kind may help distinguish movement effects caused by LBP from fatigue effects.[42]

EMG Methods of Assessing Fatigue

Surface EMG techniques for measuring fatigue in paraspinal muscles have provided a new means to objectively quantify fatigue. Before the recent technical advances in EMG acquisition and processing, most EMG studies of the back were kinesiological attempts to relate back muscle activity to different postures and loads. The major single advance in applying surface EMG to localized fatigue assessment has been the quantification of changes in the EMG waveform by power spectrum analysis.[43] This technique is based on the observation that as a contraction is sustained, there is a corresponding compression in the EMG power density spectrum (Figure 7.2). Figure 7.2 demonstrates that there is an increase in the low frequency components and a decrease in the high frequency components that comprise the signal. The change in the EMG waveform is depicted in this figure as an "elongation" of the signal which can occur as the propagation velocity of the signal is slowed by a reduction in the excitability of the muscle membrane. Changes in membrane excitability have been associated with accumulation of metabolites (e.g., H^+, K^+) at the sarcolemma.[4] A number of studies have associated metabolite accumulation with impairment of muscle contractile tension.[5,6] Other processes associated with fatigue, such as changes in re-

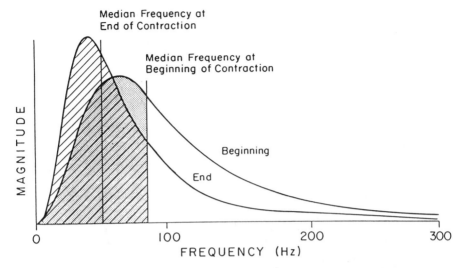

Figure 7.2 Diagram illustrating the compression of the EMG signal power density spectra from the beginning and end of a sustained contraction. The two spectra are superimposed and the median frequency of each spectrum is indicated.

cruitment of motor units[44] or changes in ionic gradients,[45] have also been shown to alter the power spectrum of the EMG waveform. Regardless of which process is present and to what degree, predictable changes in the EMG signal have been correlated with biochemical processes of fatigue. EMG can therefore be thought of as a noninvasive measure of physiological fatigue. In actuality, researchers quantify the compression of the EMG power spectrum by measuring a characteristic parameter of the spectrum such as the median or mean frequency (see Figure 7.2).[4] These parameters are computed either digitally or by specially designed analog circuits to monitor their decrease as a function of the time. The rate of decrease in mean or median frequency serves as the most common way to quantify fatigue using EMG spectral parameters. Different magnitudes of fatigue are depicted in Figure 7.3 for different percents of maximal isometric force (% MVC) which were sustained for 30 seconds by a paraspinal muscle. As expected, the higher force levels of contraction are more fatigable and result in greater changes in median frequency. Similarly, endurant muscles will have "flatter" median frequency curves (Figure 7.4).

Prior to the recent interest in using EMG spectral measures to assess fatigue in paraspinal muscle sites, most surface EMG studies were limited to a few electrode sites with analysis limited to the amplitude of the EMG signal rather than to its spectral content.[46–48] The objective of these studies was to quantify fatigue and muscle activity of the paraspinal muscles in normal

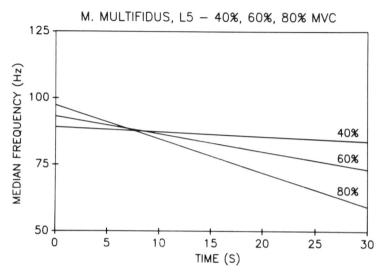

Figure 7.3 Linear regression plots for median frequency as a function of contraction duration for three different sustained force levels of contraction. Forces are expressed as a percentage of maximum (%MVC). Data is from the multifidus m. at spinal level L-5.

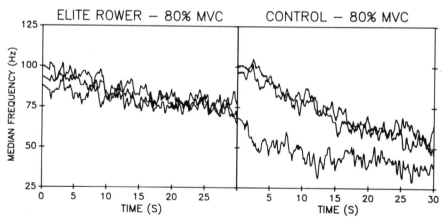

Figure 7.4 Median frequency vs. time plots from three lumbar paraspinal muscles of an elite rower compared to a sedentary control subject of approximately the same height, weight, and strength. Contractions were sustained for 30 seconds at a force level of 80%MVC.

pain-free individuals during different levels of work and in different postures. One of the earliest studies to investigate the relationship between the EMG signal and work in paraspinal muscles was performed by Morioka.[47] He reported a decrease in the EMG signal amplitude and an increase in low frequency potentials while subjects performed static lifting at 20% to 30% of their MVC. Chapman and Troup, in a similar study, observed a decrease in the total electrical activity of the muscle during the onset of fatigue symptoms.[46] They attributed this decrease in EMG to a transfer of muscle activity to other muscles of the trunk; however, in a subsequent study, the integrated EMG activity increased with fatigue.[49] They explained this inconsistency as a failure on their part to account for movements of the pelvis in their first study. Pelvic movements may have allowed slight changes in posture and thus changes in back muscle length. The need to reliably stabilize the test position is an important consideration when developing new back test procedures or evaluating existing devices and techniques. Slight changes in posture can result in a change in the pattern of muscle activation which can make data unreliable.

Back muscle endurance has also been studied during incremented static work sustained until the onset of muscular pain.[48] Paraspinal EMG was recorded bilaterally from the fourth lumbar vertebral level while subjects were placed in slight trunk flexion. The EMG signal initially increased with fatigue and then decreased during the later stages of the contraction. It was suggested that this change in the EMG was attributable to subjects altering their posture to alleviate muscle pain. This was one of the first studies to report a change in the EMG power density spectrum of lower back muscles. The low frequency components of the EMG power density spectrum increased consistently throughout the contraction in this study. The primary importance of this study was the demonstration that back pain and fatigue resulted in a consistent change in muscle activation in individuals without an LBP history. Another important early work was reported by Andersson and coworkers who used bipolar surface EMG electrodes applied to significantly more paraspinal locations than previous studies (bilateral vertebral levels T-4, T-8, L-1, L-3, and L-5).[50] In addition to studying the effects of trunk angle and load on muscle activity, they also reported that increases in EMG activity associated with trunk flexion and loading were accompanied by an increase in the rate of change of the EMG power spectrum. This study is undoubtedly among the first to include rate of spectral compression as a measure of back muscle fatigue.

The use of EMG spectral parameters to measure the rate of fatigue in back muscles from a normal subject population was investigated further by Kondraske and coworkers.[51] Their study evaluated strategies for applications of these techniques to lumbar muscles. They carried out a two-phase study in which Phase I preliminarily identified the most appropriate EMG measures of fatigue, refined test measurement procedures, established initial norms, and measured population variability and test-retest repeatability for the measures selected. Phase II was a more comprehensive evaluation of methods that was based in part on the results of Phase I. Phase II also tested the hypothesis, arising from the Phase I study, that torque expressed as a percentage of body weight is preferable to percentage MVC measures when expressing spectral shifts versus load relationships. A test frame was used to measure isometric flexion and extension torques during standing with knees flexed approximately 10 to 15 degrees. Improvements in pelvic and lower limb stabilization and force feedback were incorporated into the device for Phase II testing. Mean and median frequency parameters for monitoring spectral compression were calculated. A number of interesting findings were reported. Overall, their data suggested that the fatigue rates of trunk extensor and flexor muscles were repeatable, but the technique warranted further testing as a clinical tool. In terms of specific findings, they concluded that: (1) mean and median frequency results were comparable; (2) rate of spectral shift, although exponential, could be accurately measured by the slope of a linear regression line for a portion of the data; (3) maximum subject stabilization and analog force feedback were recommended; and (4) percent body weight was a more suitable measure of target load level than percent MVC. Their last conclusion raises an important question of whether it is appropriate to normalize contractions with respect to MVC because voluntary effort is subject to variability attributable to motivation. This concern may be even more critical for tests conducted among subjects with LBP. It is still debatable whether normalization to body weight is a solution to this problem because body weight has been shown to be a poor predictor of back muscle strength. Biederman has addressed some of these issues by implementing a technique used initially by our group in which subjects generate a constant load to the lower back by holding a specified weight at arm's length in front of them.[52] Biederman added a reference frame to standardize the position of the subject's feet, pelvis, and spine. The reliability of the technique was evaluated in 31 subjects by having them perform the weight-lifting test for 45 seconds and then repeating the test 5 days later. Paraspinal EMG signals from bilateral locations at L-2/L-3 and L-4/L-5 vertebral levels were analyzed and the root mean square (RMS) and the median frequency of the EMG signal were calculated. Reliability of EMG parameters was within an acceptable range with Pearson's correlation coefficients of $r = 0.89$ for RMS and $r = 0.85$ for median frequency. The acceptance of the technique by chronic back pain patients was also described.

Comparisons of muscle endurance measurements for low back pain patients and control subjects have also been reported in a few studies. DeVries compared chronic low back pain patients with normal control subjects during prolonged stance.[54] Subjects developing pain during the experiment showed increased paraspinal EMG activity, whereas those who experienced no pain had decreased EMG activity. Similar results were reported by Jayasinghe et al. from bilateral sacrospinalis muscles at spinal levels L-4 and L-5.[55]

They concluded that muscle weakness or fatigue is associated with low back pain. Mayer et al. reported somewhat equivocal results in their attempts to use EMG spectral analysis for endurance assessment in normal subjects and deconditioned patients.[56] Ten industrial patients undergoing functional restoration for chronic disabling spinal disorders and eleven healthy volunteers were tested by an EMG protocol combined with a Roman Chair exercise. The Roman Chair exercise apparatus uses padded pelvic supports and adjustable calf supports to place subjects in a prone position while their upper torso is held unsupported for successive fixed time trials. In this study, subjects were required to complete two successive sessions of ten trials where each trial consisted of 15 seconds of unsupported extension followed by 10 seconds of rest. EMG signals were obtained from paraspinal muscles bilaterally at 3 cm lateral to the L-3 spinous process and were analyzed using a digital sampling technique and fast Fourier transform to calculate the average mean power frequency for the first 2 seconds of each trial. The slope of decline in mean power frequency was significantly greater in back pain subjects at initial testing then either normal subjects or back pain subjects after reconditioning. These findings indicate that the EMG spectrum shifts further and recovers more slowly for back pain subjects when compared to normals and that muscle reconditioning can result in a more normal endurance capacity as measured by the EMG parameters. The test results in this study were less successful in discriminating back pain subjects from normal controls. Six of ten patients with presumed "low endurance" (MPF negative slope > 6) were not identified by the test even though they demonstrated low trunk extensor strength on isokinetic muscle tests. The authors of this study raise a number of questions regarding the usefulness of this procedure for clinical application. Aside from the issue of discriminating ability or identifying sensitivity to low back pain, they expressed a more general concern that EMG spectral parameters may not be a true index of muscle fatigue. Their reasons for this concern include the fact that their normative data was variable and covered a wide range (including a few individuals who showed no change in MPF). As such, they argued that it could not be considered a reliable technique for identifying subjects outside of the normal range. It was postulated from these findings that fatigue may be the result of different mechanisms in different individuals. Furthermore, the investigators were troubled by the fact that in their tests the MPF declined nonlinearly and therefore a "fatigue index" based on MPF slope would be dependent on the end point of the contraction. The study raises valid questions regarding the identification of a universally applicable fatigue index and challenges the definition of fatigue. These issues are topics of intensive debate and research. Rather than negating its usefulness, it is incumbent on the community of researchers in this field to explore more carefully the development of well-controlled and standardized proce-

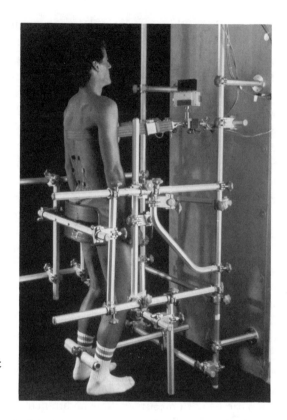

Figure 7.5 A prototype postural restraint device and force acquisition system that was used in the initial Back Analysis System (BAS).

dures. Keep in mind that the application of this technique is truly in its infancy and more effective protocols and analysis techniques are needed. New developments have met with some success in this regard according to the results of recent investigations conducted by our group and others.[57–60]

Roy and coworkers developed an EMG acquisition and processing system that includes a postural restraint device to measure isometric torques and provide visual feedback of the force produced during trunk extension.[58–60] Different versions of this system, referred to as a Back Analysis System (BAS), are depicted in Figures 7.5 and 7.6. The array of six active surface EMG electrodes on the lumbar paraspinal muscles is shown in the figures. Active electrodes refer to the fact that signal conditioning circuitry is present at or very near the detection surface, thereby minimizing the effect of skin impedance or movement of leads.[3] The locations of the surface electrodes were selected according to specific muscle groups (longissimus thoracis, ilicostalis lumborum, and multifidus) at specified vertebral levels (L-1, L-2, L-5) rather than following previously employed techniques which used fixed distances from bony landmarks as the location criteria.[56] It is our belief that it is more important to be consistent in locating a surface EMG electrode on a particular

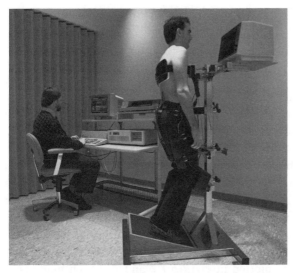

Figure 7.6 The current version of the Back Analysis System (BAS) designed for clinical as well as laboratory use. (From Roy SH, De Luca CJ, Casavant DA: Lumbar muscle fatigue and chronic lower back pain. Spine 1989; 14:994. With permission of the publisher.)

muscle group than it is to adhere to a procedure based on fixed distances. When fixed bony landmarks are used, individual differences in body size and anatomy will dictate which muscle group is detected. Without consistency in muscle detection, it may not be possible to make functional interpretations from the EMG parameters, particularly when comparisons are made across subjects. The issue of EMG signal reliability as it pertains to electrode location is discussed more fully in recent publications.[61,62] Signals from neighboring or even very distant muscles can theoretically propagate by volume conduction to the electrode site. This phenomenon, called *crosstalk*, can result in invalid findings when attempting to characterize or isolate a specific muscle group by the surface EMG signal. EMG studies of back muscles that include arrays of electrodes on different muscle groups cannot automatically be assumed to provide specific information about each of the individual muscle groups that lie directly beneath each electrode. Research to date suggests that crosstalk can be minimized by carefully selecting large superficial muscle groups and using bipolar differential electrodes with relatively small interelectrode separation (1 cm or less). Crosstalk has been measured and reported in limb muscles but not back muscles.[61,63] Preliminary work in over 50 experiments conducted by Merletti et al. resulted in much less crosstalk between superficial back muscles (longissimus thoracis and iliocostalis lumborum) than had previously been reported for muscles of the lower leg[61] and thigh.[63] It may be that the lumbodorsal fascia severely attenuates signals from neighboring muscles.

Studies using the Back Analysis System have included low back patients from sedentary[58] and athletic populations.[59,60] The reliability and validity of the Back Analysis System was first evaluated by testing male chronic low back pain patients (n = 12) and control subjects without pain (n = 12). Patients were deliberately selected to be in remission and have at least a 6-month history of LBP. It was argued that this selection criteria would increase the possibility that differences in muscular performance, if present, were the result of physiological factors rather than psychogenic factors. The study required each subject to sustain a constant force isometric contraction for a maximum of 1 minute at each of three target force levels: 40% MVC, 60% MVC, and 80% MVC. The study design included different force levels to determine which combination of muscle sites and load magnitude would provide the highest sensitivity and selectivity for LBP. It was postulated that this information would be useful for identifying the optimal protocol for the technique. The first set of findings characterized muscle behavior for normal and back pain subjects and found certain similarities and differences. The summary statistics for initial median frequency (IMF) values and median frequency slope are plotted in Figures 7.7 and 7.8. Each figure contains data for the longissimus (L-1), iliocostalis (L-2) and multifidus (L-5) muscle groups. In each plot, the data from the left and right sides of the back are further subdivided, as are the force levels of the contraction. Similarities between the two subject groups were that the IMF decreased for increasing force levels of contraction; the negative slope of the median frequency was higher as the force level of the contraction increased, particularly at the L-5 detection site. The decrease in IMF with force indicates that the Type II fibers associated with more forceful contractions have lower conduction velocities than the Type I fibers. Recall that morphological studies of paraspinal muscles describe Type II fibers as having smaller cross-sectional areas than Type I fibers,[12–14] which could account for these findings because EMG conduction velocity is proportional to the muscle cross-sectional area.[3,4] The increase in the negative slope of the median frequency with increased force is consistent with numerous findings from limb muscles[3,4] which indicate that Type II fibers recruited at high force levels accumulate metabolites at a high rate and thereby accelerate the compression of the EMG spectrum. The differences in the median frequency parameters for the three lumbar levels may be directly related to differences in mechanical advantage and other biomechanical factors that determine the amount of force a muscle needs to produce to generate a particular extension moment. The higher median frequency slope observed at L-5 is consistent with biomechanical studies that describe proportionately higher forces for lower lumbar muscles than for upper lumbar muscles.[64]

Differences in EMG median frequency between normal and back pain subjects are also summarized in Figures 7.7 and 7.8. The data from low back pain subjects exhibited significantly higher median frequency slopes than

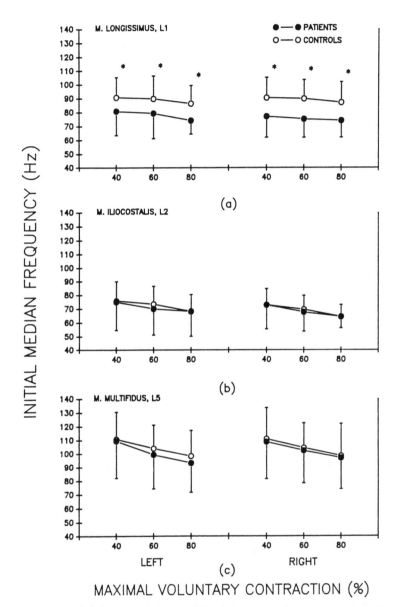

Figure 7.7 Mean initial median frequency for left and right muscle groups for three %MVC forces tested in patients (●) and control (O) subjects. Plots are presented for the (a) longissimus (L-1), (b) iliocostalis (L-2), and (c) multifidus (L-5) muscles. *P < 0.05 for significance of difference between means. [From Roy SH, De Luca CJ, Casavant DA: Lumbar muscle fatigue and chronic lower back pain. Spine 1989; 14:997. With permission of the publisher.]

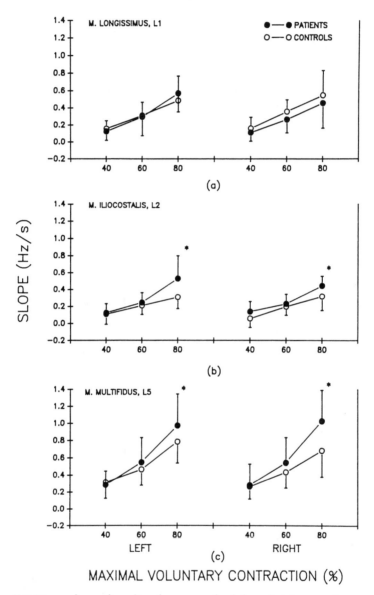

Figure 7.8 Mean slope of median frequency for left and right muscle groups for three %MVC forces tested in patients (●) and control (O) subjects. Plots are presented for the (a) longissimus (L1), (b) iliocostalis (L2), and (c) multifidus (L5) muscles. *P < 0.05 for significance of difference between means. (From Roy SH, De Luca CJ, Casavant DA: Lumbar muscle fatigue and chronic lower back pain. Spine 1989; 14:997. With permission of the publisher.)

control subjects at 80% MVC for the L-2 and L-5 muscle groups. This finding is consistent with other studies which conclude that back pain subjects on average have more fatigable back muscles than normal pain-free individuals.[32,37,54,55] A second possible interpretation of these results is that some back muscles may contribute a proportionately greater component of force than other back muscles and therefore develop higher levels of fatigue. Because not all muscle sites or load levels differed significantly between LBP patients and controls, it appears that median frequency behavior is muscle dependent as well as load specific. The results of this study indicate that high levels of contraction and inclusion of lower lumbar muscle sites should be considered as important components of EMG studies that attempt to differentiate muscle function in LBP patients from normal back muscle function.

Initial median frequency values for L-1 muscle sites were significantly lower in the LBP patient group compared to the control group independent of %MVC or side studied. No such differences were reported for L-2 or L-5 muscle sites. Considering that the median frequency estimate is proportional to the average cross-sectional area of the muscle fibers, the authors postulate that this result may indicate that chronic LBP patients have generalized muscle atrophy associated with disuse. It would be speculative at this time to offer an explanation as to why this effect was present in the upper lumbar area and not the lower lumbar region. However, the answer may be tied to the observation from our group (unpublished) that the most striking difference between highly trained and novice rowers is the increased activation and improved endurance capacity of the upper compared to lower lumbar muscles as measured by EMG median frequency parameters. These findings imply that more attention may need to be directed toward conditioning upper back muscles. Unless challenged by intensive exercises focused on the upper lumbar and mid-thoracic paraspinals, these regions probably do not receive sufficient activation to see a training effect. The sedentary nature of our lifestyle probably contributes further to this deconditioning process. Biomechanical models of paraspinal muscle forces have indicated much higher levels of tension in lower lumbar muscles than upper lumbar or thoracic muscles.[64] Loads normally encountered in daily activities may be sufficient to keep lower lumbar muscles properly activated but not upper lumbar spinal musculature. The implication of this finding is that strengthening and endurance activities should involve the upper extremities so that scapular and mid-thoracic trunk musculature can be recruited. Reliance only on dynamometers that isolate the lower back and eliminate the use of the arms for transference of load to the upper back may therefore be inadequate for reconditioning. The fact that back muscles are almost always loaded via manual tasks during work hardening programs may explain in part why this type of

Table 7.2   Results from Discriminant Analyses for LBP Using BAS Data from Separate Lumbar Levels

Lumbar Level	Force Level (%MVC)	Correct Classification		Discriminant Variables (in order)
		Normal	LBP	
L1	80	8/12	8/11	(L) IMF
	60	8/12	9/12	(R) IMF, (L) SLOPE
	40	8/12	9/12	(R) IMF, (L) SLOPE
L2	80	10/12	8/12	(L) SLOPE, (R) SLOPE
	40	9/12	8/12	(R) SLOPE, (L) SLOPE
L5	80	9/12	19/12	(R) SLOPE, (L) IMF
	60	9/12	6/12	(R) SLOPE

Abbreviations: (R), (L), right side, left side; LBP, low back pain; IMF, initial median frequency; SLOPE, median frequency slope.

program is meeting with some success in reconditioning trunk musculature to meet the functional demands of the spine.

The sensitivity and specificity of median frequency estimates to identify individuals with low back pain were also evaluated by our group [58-60] as well as others.[53] In a case/control study of chronic back pain subjects, we entered the median frequency parameters, consisting of slope and initial values of median frequency, into a two-group, stepwise discriminant analysis procedure. Discriminant analysis is a multivariate statistical procedure that identifies which combination of variables is most effective at separating the subject population into specified groups. The results of the discriminant analysis are presented in Tables 7.2 and 7.3. A maximum of six noncorrelated variables were entered into this discriminant analysis procedure. Table 7.3 summarizes the results from the analysis in which data from all muscle sites were entered into the analysis; separate analyses were conducted for the 40%, 60%, and 80% MVC trials. The best classification results corresponded to trials conducted at 40% MVC and 80% MVC. No more than two false positive or false negative classifications resulted. Performance suffered somewhat for the 60% MVC trials, particularly for identification of control subjects. It may be that muscle deficits are more apparent at the extremes of the contractile force range where disproportionate fiber types are likely to be present. The variables entered into the classification functions were primarily the initial median frequency (IMF) from L-1 and the median frequency slope at L-2 and/or L-5. A comparison of results between Table 7.2 and Table 7.3 demonstrates a higher percentage of correct classification for analysis in which all electrode sites are included in the discriminant analysis than for the analysis in which muscle groups are treated separately. This result fur-

Table 7.3 Results from Discriminant Analyses for LBP Using BAS Data from All Lumbar Levels

Force Level (%MVC)	Correct Classification		Discriminant Variables (in order)
	Normal	LBP	
40	11/12	9/11	(R) IMF, L1
			(R) SLOPE, L2
			(L) SLOPE, L2
			(L) SLOPE, L1
			(L) IMF, L1
60	8/12	9/12	(R) IMF, L1
			(L) SLOPE, L1
80	10/12	10/11	(L) IMF, L1
			(R) SLOPE, L5
			(L) SLOPE, L2

Abbreviations: (R), (L), right side, left side; LBP, low back pain; IMF, initial median frequency; SLOPE, median frequency slope.

ther supports the postulate that arrays of electrodes, rather than a few bilateral sites, provide the most accurate results. The limited success of past EMG studies involving back muscles and LBP may have been due in part to this factor.

The successful implementation of the EMG signal procedures described above for chronic LBP subjects led us to investigate whether the technique could correctly identify individuals with LBP within a population of elite athletes.[59,60] We were interested in determining whether athletes with LBP might have a muscular component to their back disorder despite the fact that they are highly conditioned. This objective raises the larger question of whether different kinds of muscular disturbances can be present and whether these differences are measurable by one technique. There may be recognizable patterns of EMG signals for specific kinds of disorders or within specific populations of individuals.

Twenty-three members of a men's collegiate varsity crew team consisting of port (n = 13) and starboard (n = 10) rowers were tested using the Back Analysis System previously described. Six of the rowers tested were further classified as having low back pain. Because our previous study on chronic LBP subjects indicated that contractions sustained at 80% MVC were most effective at identifying muscle deficits associated with LBP, we limited the test procedures to this one contraction level. Contractions were sustained for a duration of 30 seconds. In addition to monitoring EMG spectral change associated with fatigue, recovery from fatigue was also included in the protocol and analysis. A "recovery" contraction (80% MVC × 5s) was conducted 1 minute following the 30 second sustained contraction. The percent recovery of MF at 1 minute (REC) was calculated from the ratio:

$$REC (\%) = [IMF2 - FMF1] / [IMF1 - FMF1] \times 100\%$$

where:

IMF1 is the initial MF of the 80% MVC × 30s contraction;
FMF1 is the final MF of the 80% MVC × 30s contraction; and
IMF2 is the initial MF of the 80% MVC × 10s contraction.

Basically, this parameter expresses the degree to which the median frequency has returned to its baseline, prefatigued value as a result of a 1 minute rest following the fatigue-inducing contraction. It was felt that the recovery parameter would be a useful measure of the ability of a muscle to recover from metabolite accumulation following strenuous exercise.

A two-group discriminant analysis for LBP and non-LBP categories resulted in 100% correct classification of the LBP rowers and 93% correct classification of non-LBP rowers (one false positive identification). Variables used in the classification function were primarily the recovery parameters (REC) from L-5 and L-1 electrode locations. None of the parameters used to classify LBP and non-LBP individuals from our previous study on sedentary chronic LBP patients were used in this group of elite rowers. This finding is not surprising considering that the differences in IMF and MF slope among nonathletes was most likely indicative of muscle disuse. Disuse would not be likely among rowers with LBP because they continued to be involved in training and competition to the same extent as their non-LBP counterparts. The fact that recovery was such a strong discriminator for LBP in this population may be a reflection of the unique energy requirements of the sport of rowing. During competition, rowers quickly achieve a marked anaerobic response and must tolerate high levels of excessive lactate throughout the remainder of the race.[65] It is possible that the inefficient physiological removal of these high levels of lactate is a sequela of LBP in rowers. The implication of this finding is that rowers with LBP may need to emphasize recovery from fatigue in their training regimens.

Direct comparisons between the methods incorporated into the BAS analysis and standard clinical assessment of the lower back and trunk have been conducted. Klein and coworkers recruited 25 freshman rowers for this study, 8 of whom had a history of chronic LBP.[60] Protocols similar to those described previously for the BAS were conducted on all subjects. In addition, each subject was evaluated for trunk and spinal mobility using conventional clinical procedures as well as maximal isometric strength during trunk extension (using the BAS restraint device). A two-group stepwise discriminant analysis procedure for the ROM and MVC variables correctly identified 57% of the LBP rowers and 63% of the non-LBP rowers. A similar discriminant analysis procedure for EMG spectral parameters correctly identified 100% of the LBP rowers and 88% of the non-LBP rowers. The high sensitivity and specificity of the latter technique indicates that it may be superior to conventional clinical measures of trunk mobility and strength for LBP screening or diagnosis.

Other investigations of back muscle fatigue by EMG spectral analysis studied the discriminating ability of spectral parameters to distinguish between normal controls and LBP patients classified according to a Pain Behavior Checklist.[53] This scale categorizes back pain patients into "confronter" and "avoider" groups based on their behavioral response to back pain.[66] It is postulated that these categories reflect the clinical observation that some patients remain very active despite their reported back problems, whereas others tend to avoid physical and social activities as much as possible to protect their painful condition. Based on this classification, the avoiders had consistently higher pain scores and a lower level of physical mobility than the confronters. The data were analyzed using a two-part procedure whereby a canonical discriminant analysis was first conducted to identify the parameters that would best discriminate between the groups. The discriminant functions from this analysis were then used to reclassify subjects. This procedure resulted in 88.9% correct identification of avoiders; one case was misclassified as a member of the confronter group. There was also a considerable amount of overlap between confronters and normals which may indicate a high degree of functional similarity between the two groups. Of the parameters contributing most to the discriminant functions, it was found that they were primarily from lower lumbar paraspinals (multifidus, L-4, -5) rather than the upper lumbar areas (iliocostalis lumborum, L-2, -3). The median frequency slope was a key component of the discriminant function accounting for the highest percentage of the variance between the three groups. Furthermore, the median frequency slope of the avoider patient group was twice as high (more negative) as the confronter group or control group. There appeared to be a continuum of fatigue rates with the avoider patient group having the highest mean value, the controls the lowest, and the confronter patient group intermediately located. Based on these findings, the authors of this study postulated that the avoider patient group may have a compromised endurance capacity resulting from either a lower ratio of slow twitch to fast twitch muscle fibers or a degenerative process involving the Type I slow twitch muscle fibers. The development of these muscle characteristics was viewed as either an adaptive response to changes in functional demand or genetic variations which could put certain people at higher risk of LBP.

Conclusion

This review summarized the role of muscle fatigue in normal spinal function and LBP. It is apparent from the studies cited that muscle dysfunction is an important component to LBP disorders. The ability of the trunk musculature to maintain adequate levels of tension demanded by a particular task may rapidly degrade if fatigue processes are present. There is evidence, though not conclusive, that muscle fatigue alters the kinematics and kinetics of the trunk which can predispose the musculoskeletal tissue to injury. Most of the evidence for associating fatigue with muscle injury is indirect. For instance, retrospective studies have related LBP to occupations that are characterized by inducing muscular fatigue.

New instrumentation for trunk assessment has advanced our ability to address the relationship between muscle fatigue and muscle injury more directly. Objective techniques for assessing muscle fatigue are no longer limited to limb musculature. Back dynamometers are available for studying isometric, isokinetic, and isoinertial contractions. Protocols developed for these instruments are beginning to include measurements of endurance. Many of these systems were previously limited to strength assessment or purely static modes. Now it is possible to measure how torque production changes with velocity or displacement in either single or multiple planes simultaneously. Changes in the interrelationship between these parameters during fatigue or as a result of LBP may provide a more dynamic measure of spine function than do conventional techniques.

The technique of surface electromyography is just beginning to emerge from the research laboratory into the LBP clinic. Advances in our knowledge of the physiological basis for EMG signal modification coupled with improved instrumentation for its measurement has made this technique a viable complement to existing procedures of back assessment.

Combined, the dynamometer and EMG techniques of back assessment may provide researchers and clinicians with new ways of defining what is meant by "normal" spine function. Before this information can be used diagnostically, more research is needed to develop normative data bases that take into consideration such factors as age, occupation, and gender. Identification of how the neuromuscular system adapts to either acute or chronic LBP has also progressed, but many questions remain. One of the greatest challenges facing the researcher and clinician today is to demonstrate the clinical efficacy of techniques that measure muscle fatigability. This task is particularly challenging for LBP assessment and treatment. More prospective, randomized blind studies need to be performed in the future to validate the relevance of fatigue measurements to clinical outcome and function.

References

1. Frymoyer JW, Gordon SL (ed): New Perspective on Low Back Pain. American Academy of Orthopedic Surgeons, Illinois, 1989.
2. White A A III, Gordon SL: Synopsis: Workshop on idiopathic low back pain. Spine 7:141–149, 1982.
3. Basmajian JV, De Luca CJ: Muscles Alive. Baltimore, Williams and Wilkins, 1985.
4. De Luca CJ: Myoelectric manifestation of localized muscular fatigue in humans. CRC Critical Reviews in Biomedical Engineering 11(4): 251–279, 1985.
5. Maclaren DPM, Gibson H, Parry-Billings M, Edwards RHT: A review of metabolic and physiological factors in fatigue. Exerc Sports Sci Rev 17:29–66, 1989.
6. Kirkendal DT: Mechanisms of peripheral fatigue. Med Sci Sports Exerc, 22(4): 444–449, 1990.
7. Brooks GA, Fahey TD: Exercise Physiology: Human Bioenergetics and Its Applications. New York, MacMillian, 1985.
8. Astrand P, Rudahl K: Textbook of Work Physiology. New York, McGraw-Hill, 1986.
9. Shultz A, Haderspeck K, Warwick D, Portillo D: Use of Lumbar trunk muscles in isometric performance of mechanically complex standing tasks. J Orthop Res, 1(1): 77–91, 1983.
10. Garrett W, Bradley W, Byrd S, Edgerton VR, Gollnick P: Basic Science Perspective. In Frymoyer JW, Gordon SL (ed): New Perspectives on Low Back Pain. IL, American Academy of Orthopaedic Surgeons, 1989.
11. Sulemena CA, Suclenwirth R: Topische Unterschiede in der enzymhistologischen zusamm ensetzung der skelettmuskilatur. J Neurol Sci 16: 433–444, 1972.
12. Sirca A, Kostevc V: The fiber type composition of thoracic and lumbar paravertebral muscles in man. J Anat 141:131–137, 1985.
13. Bagnall KM, Ford DM, McFadden KD, Greenhill BJ, Raso VJ: The histochemical composition of human vertebral muscle. Spine 9:470–473, 1984.
14. Ford D, Bagnall KM, McFadden KD, Greenhill B, Raso VJ: Analysis of vertebral muscle obtained during surgery for correction of a lumbar disc disorder. Acta Anatomica 116:152–157, 1983.
15. Fidler MW, Jowett RL, Troup JDG: Myosin ATPase activity in multifidus muscle from cases of lumbar spinal derangement. J Bone Joint Surg 57-B:220–227, 1975.
16. Musacchia XJ, Steffen JM, Fell RD: Disuse atrophy of skeletal muscle: Animal models. In Pandolph KB (ed): Exercise and Sports Science Reviews, 16:61–87, MacMillan, 1988.

17. Edgerton VR, Roy RR: Adaptations of skeletal muscle to spaceflight. In Churchill S (ed): Fundamentals of Space Life Sciences, Cambridge, MA, MIT Press, 1990.

18. Seidel H, Beyer H, Brauer D: Electromyographic evaluation of back muscle fatigue with repeated sustained contraction of different strengths. Eur J Appl Physiol 56:592–602, 1987.

19. Dupuis H, Zerlett G: Whole-body vibration and disorder of the spine. Int Arch Occup Environ Health 59:323–336, 1987.

20. Bigos SJ, Battie MC: Surveillance of back problems in industry. In Hadler NM (ed): Clinical Concepts in Regional Musculoskeletal Illness. Orlando, Grune and Stratton, 99–315, 1987.

21. Brewer BJ: Mechanism of injury to the musculotendinous unit. In Reynold FC (ed): American Academy of Orthopaedic Surgeons Instructional Course Lectures, XVII. St. Louis, Mosby, 354–358, 1960.

22. Tidball JG: Myotendinous junction: Morphological changes and mechanical failure associated with muscle cell atrophy. Exp Mol Pathol 40:1–12, 1984.

23. Edgerton VR, Bodine SC, Roy RR: Muscle architecture and performance: Stress and strain relationship in a muscle with two compartments arranged in series. In Marconnet P, Komi PV (eds): Muscular Function in Exercise and Training. Basal, S Karger, 26:12–23, 1987.

24. Wiktorsson-Moller M, Oberg R, Ekstrand J, et al: Effects of warm-up, massage, and stretching on range of motion and muscle strength in the lower extremity. Am J Sports Med 4:124–128, 1983.

25. Ekstrand J, Gillquist J: The avoidability of soccer injuries. Int J Sports Med 4:124–128, 1983.

26. Garrett WE Jr, Safran MR, Seaber AV, et al: Biomechanical comparison of stimulated and nonstimulated skeletal muscle pulled to failure. Am J Sports Med 15:452, 1987.

27. Safran MR, Garrett WE Jr, Seaber AV, et al: The role of warm-up in muscular injury prevention. Am J Sports Med 16:123–129, 1988.

28. Sapega AA, Sokolow DP, Graham TJ, Chance B: Phosphorus nuclear magnetic resonance: A non-invasive technique for the study of muscle bioenergetics during exercise. Med Sci Sports Exerc 19(4): 410–42, 1987.

29. Nordin M, Kahanovitz N, Verderame R, et al: Normal trunk muscle strength and endurance in women and the effect of exercises and electrical stimulation, Part I: Normal endurance and trunk muscle strength in 101 women. Spine 12:105–111, 1987.

30. Nicolaisen T, Jorgensen K: Trunk strength, back muscle endurance and low-back trouble. Scand J Rehabil Med 17:121–127, 1985.

31. Biering-Sorensen F: Physical measurements as risk indication for low back trouble over a one-year period. Spine 9:106–119, 1984.

32. Jorgensen K, Nicolaisen T: Trunk extensor endurance: Determination and relation to low-back trouble. Ergonomics 30:259–267, 1987.

33. Smidt G, Herring T, Amundsen L, et al: Assessment of abdominal and back extensor function: A quantitative approach and results for chronic low-back patients. Spine 8:211–219, 1983.

34. Hasue M, Fujiwara J, Kikuchi S: A new method of quantitative measurements of abdominal and back muscle strength. Spine 5:142–148, 1980.

35. Parnianpour M, Nordin M, Kahanovitz N, Frankel V, Kahanovitz N: The triaxial coupling of torque generation of trunk muscles during isometric exertions and the effect of fatiguing isoinertial movements on the motor output and movement patterns. Spine 13(9): 982–992, 1988.

36. Hansen JW: Postoperative management in lumbar disc protrusions. Acta Orthop Scand (suppl) 71:1–47, 1964.

37. Nicolaisen T, Jorgensen K: Trunk strength, back muscle endurance and low-back trouble. Scand J Rehabil Med 17:121–127, 1985.

38. Jorgensen K, Nicolaisen T: Two methods for determining trunk extensor endurance: A comparative study. Eur J Appl Physiol 55:639–644, 1986.

39. Jorgensen K: Back muscle strength and body weight as limiting factors for work in the standing slightly-stooped position. Scand J Rehab Med 2:149–153, 1970.

40. Seeds RH, Levene JA, Goldberg HM: Abnormal patient data for the Isostation B100. J Orth Sports Phys Ther 10(4): 121–133, 1988.

41. Levene JA, Seeds RH, Goldberg HM, Frazier M, Fuhrman GA: Trends in isodynamic and isometric trunk testing on the Isostation B-200. J Spinal Disorders 2(1): 20–35, 1989.

42. McIntyre DR, Glover LH: Secondary axes activity of normal subjects and low back pain patients. In press.

43. Merletti R, De Luca CJ: New techniques in surface electromyography. In Desmedt JE (ed): Computer Aided Electromyography and Expert Systems, Elsevier Science Publisher B.V., 1989.

44. Solomonow M, Baratta R, Baten C, Smit J, Hermens H, D'Ambrosia RD: Electromyogram power spectra frequencies associated with motor unit recruitment strategies. J Appl Physiol 68(3): 1177, 1990.

45. Juel C: Muscle action potential propagation velocity changes during activity. Muscle and Nerve 1:714–719, 1988.

46. Chapman AE, Troup JD: Prolonged activity of lumbar erectores spinae: An electromyographic and dynamometric study of the effect of training. Ann Phys Med 10:262–269, 1970.

47. Morioka M: Some physiologic responses to the static muscular exercises. Rep Inst Sci Labour 63:6–24, 1964.

48. Okada M, Kogi K, Ishii M: Enduring capacity of the erectores spinae in static work. J Anthrop Soc Nippon 78:99–110, 1970.

49. Troup JD, Chapman AE: Changes in the waveform of the electromyogram during fatiguing activity in the muscles of the spine and hips: The analysis of postural stress. Electromyogr Clin Neurophysiol 12:347–365, 1972.

50. Andersson GBJ, Ortengren R, Herberts P: Quantitative electromyographic studies of back muscle activity related to posture and loading. Orthop Clin North Am 8:85–96, 1977.

51. Kondraske GV, Carmichael T, Mayer TG, Deivanayagam S, Mooney V: Myoelectric spectral analysis and strategies for quantifying trunk muscular fatigue. Arch Phys Med Rehabil 68:103–110, 1987.

52. Biederman HJ: Weight-lifting in a postural restraining device: A reliable method to generate paraspinal constant-force contraction. Clin Biomed, in press.

53. Biederman HJ, Shanks GL, Inglis J: Median frequency estimates of paraspinal muscles: Reliability analysis. Electromyog Clin Neurophys, in press.

54. DeVries HA: EMG fatigue curves in postural muscles: A possible etiology for idiopathic low back pain. Am J Phys Med 47:175–181, 1968.

55. Jayasinghe WJ, Harding RH, Anderson JAD, Sweetman BJ: An electromyographic investigation of postural fatigue in low back pain: A preliminary study. Electroencephalog Clin Neurophysiol 18:191–198, 1978.

56. Mayer TG, Kondraske G, Mooney V, Carmichael TW, Butsch R: Lumbar myoelectric spectral analysis for endurance assessment: A comparison of normals with deconditioned patients. Spine 14(9): 986–991, 1989.

57. Merletti R, Lo Conte LR, Orizio C: Indices of muscle fatigue. J Electromy Kines 1(1): 20–33, 1991.

58. Roy SH, De Luca CJ, Casavant DA: Lumbar muscle fatigue and chronic low back pain. Spine 14(9): 992–1001, 1989.

59. Roy SH, De Luca CJ, Snyder-Mackler L, Emley MS, Crenshaw RL, Lyons J P: Fatigue, recovery and low back pain in varsity rowers. Med Sci Sports Exerc 22(4): 463–469, 1990.

60. Klein AB, Snyder-Mackler L, Roy SH, De Luca CJ: Comparison of spinal mobility and isometric trunk extensor strength to EMG spectral analysis in identifying low back pain. Physical Therapy 71(6): 445–454, 1991.

61. Merletti R, De Luca CJ: Crosstalk in surface electromyography. In Desmedt JE (ed): Computer-Aided Electromyography and Expert Systems. Elsevier Science Publisher BV, 1989.

62. Roy SH, De Luca CJ, Schneider J: Effects of electrode location on myoelectric conduction velocity and median frequency estimates. J Appl Physiol 61:1510–1517, 1986.

63. Emley M, Catani F, Roy SH, Knaflitz M: Myoelectric crosstalk in antagonist muscles of the human thigh. Proc IEEE-EMBS 9th Ann Int Conf, Boston, 1987.

64. Yettram AL, Bai BA, Jackman MJ: Equilibrium analysis for the forces in the human spinal column and its musculature. Spine 5:402–411, 1980.
65. Hagerman FC, Conors MC, Gault JA, Hagerman GR, Polinski WJ: Energy expenditure during simulated rowing. J Appl Physiol 45:87–93, 1971.
66. Zarkowska AW: The relationship between subjective behavioral aspects of pain in people suffering from lower back pain. M Phil, University of London, 1981.

8

□ □ □
□ □ □
□ □ □

Advancements in Functional Capacity Evaluation

Susan J. Isernhagen

History and Present Use

The Problem to the Medical Community

Historically, one variable affecting significantly rising costs in work injury management is the slow process of returning injured workers to work. Costs associated with the delayed process include both financial ones, such as Worker's Compensation, loss of productivity, replacement of the injured worker, and human costs of disability, functional loss, and deprivation of worker identity.

In the late 1970s, Worker's Compensation administrations became alarmed at these rising costs. They began to look for the cause of delay in "the system." While there were many confounding factors, a primary delay identified was lack of specific "release to work" information by the physician. In some cases, the physician was hesitant to identify when a worker could return to work. In other cases, releases were often written in vague terms such as "5 pound lifting restrictions," or "light duty only." This lack of definitive evaluation blocked the rehabilitation consultant or the employer from finding specific work for an injured worker. In addition, workers themselves were unsure of their own physical abilities.

To improve the situation, a form was developed that required more specific information about actual physical abilities of the worker (see Figure 8.1). States and insurance companies used the same format, asking for estimated functional capacities. This form not only included the amount of heavy physical work (lifting, carrying) but also listed other important aspects of work such as sitting, standing, walking, bending, crouching, and so on that are as critical for employability as lifting capacity.

**WORKERS COMPENSATION
FUNCTIONAL CAPACITY FORM**

PATIENT:_____

I would estimate this person to be able to:

		Never	Occasionally (1-33%)	Frequently (34-66%)	Continuously (67-100%)
1.	LIFT:				
	a. up to 10#	_____	_____	_____	_____
	b. 11 - 25#	_____	_____	_____	_____
	c. 26 - 35#	_____	_____	_____	_____
	d. 36 - 50#	_____	_____	_____	_____
	e. 51 - 75#	_____	_____	_____	_____
	f. 76 - 100#	_____	_____	_____	_____
2.	CARRY:				
	a. up to 10#	_____	_____	_____	_____
	b. 11 - 25#	_____	_____	_____	_____
	c. 26 - 34#	_____	_____	_____	_____
	d. 36 - 50#	_____	_____	_____	_____
	e. 51 - 75#	_____	_____	_____	_____
	f. 76 - 100#	_____	_____	_____	_____

3.   CAN THE PERSON PERFORM
   THE FOLLOWING TASKS:

	Never	Occasionally	Frequently	Continuously
Push/Pull - seated	_____	_____	_____	_____
Push/Pull-standing	_____	_____	_____	_____
Bend	_____	_____	_____	_____
Squat	_____	_____	_____	_____
Crawl	_____	_____	_____	_____
Climb	_____	_____	_____	_____
Reach above shoulder level	_____	_____	_____	_____

4.   CIRCLE THE NUMBER OF HOURS FOR EACH ACTIVITY:
   Note: Does not have to total 8 hours.

		Continually	With Rests
Sit	1 2 3 4 5 6 7 8 (hours)	_____	_____
Stand	1 2 3 4 5 6 7 8 (hours)	_____	_____
Walk	1 2 3 4 5 6 7 8 (hours)	_____	_____
Sit/Stand	1 2 3 4 5 6 7 8 (hours)	_____	_____

A

Figure 8.1 The workers compensation functional capacity form requires more specific information about actual physical abilities of the worker.

It is important to note that this form was made for estimates, not specificity. For example, the type of lifting is not defined, even though lifting ability is directly related to the level of the lift (floor level, knuckle level, overhead, etc.). This form encourages generalities in estimating the maxi-

SAMPLE WORKERS COMPENSATION FUNCTIONAL CAPACITY FORM

5.   CAN PERSON USE HANDS FOR REPETITIVE ACTION SUCH AS:

	Simple Grasping	Firm Grasp	Fine Manipulating
Right	Yes____ No____	Yes____ No____	Yes____ No____
Left	Yes____ No____	Yes____ No____	Yes____ No____

SAME WORKERS COMPENSATION FUNCTIONAL CAPACITY FORM

6.   CAN PERSON USE FEET FOR REPETITIVE MOVEMENTS, AS IN OPERATING FOOT CONTROLS?

Right	Left	Both
Yes____ No____	Yes____ No____	Yes____ No____

7.   ANY RESTRICTIONS OF ACTIVITIES INVOLVED?

8.   CAN PERSON NOW RETURN TO FORMER JOB?

Yes____   No____

CAN PERSON RETURN TO OTHER WORK ACCORDING TO RESTRICTIONS DEFINED ABOVE?

Yes____   No____

IF NOT, GIVE ESTIMATED DATE FOR RETURN TO WORK_____

Work part-time? ____hrs/day Work full-time? Yes____ No____
Disability rating _____& (if applicable)

9.   COMMENTS:_____

_____

_____

_____

_____

_____

_____

_____   _____
          Physician   Date

B

Figure 8.1 (continued)

mum capacity of lift (25 to 40 pounds), even though the maximum function is measurable. The "frequency of work" categories match the *Dictionary of Occupational Titles* in defining the portion of a day that an activity is performed. Therefore, the estimated functional capacity form serves the purpose of asking the evaluator to think both in functional terms and also in regard to an 8-hour work day.

The Challenge

Although physicians have been designated as gatekeepers of the injured worker case, they have not traditionally been work evaluators. On the other hand, physical and occupational therapists have traditionally evaluated function, understand pathology, spend time with the client, and are equipped by education to perform tests such as functional capacity evaluations (FCE). They are now considered the professionals of choice as FCE comprehensive evaluators.[1-4]

When the therapist performs an FCE, specific return-to-work performance is measured. In addition to assisting medical release, the comprehensive evaluation allows the workers to feel more confident about their own abilities because they actually have been "tested." The information provides accuracy and expediency of return-to-work information for both the physician and the worker. The employer then has usable, nonadversarial information with which to place the worker at work.

A Test of Function, Not of the Job

How does the therapist decide what should be included in an FCE? In reviewing Figure 8.1 it is clear that this requires an evaluation of a person in relationship to work activities. The questions do not initially relate to a worker's job, but rather to the worker specifically. For example, if a worker, Clarence Peterson, is being considered for release to return to work, the physician and employer must know Clarence's physical abilities. Once a functional capacity evaluation is performed, the employer can match Clarence's abilities against the critical demands of the job. If there is a match, then Clarence can return to work. If there is not a match, then there are three options:

1. modifying the original job;
2. matching Clarence to a different job;
3. rehabilitating Clarence.

Because an evaluation is person specific, Clarence's abilities can be compared to an unlimited number of jobs. Also, the definition of Clarence's limitations allows specific modifications. If rehabilitation is required, Clarence's deficiencies will be noted and a rehabilitation plan can be made matching the physical deficiencies to appropriate rehabilitation techniques. This makes the rehabilitation plan specific to Clarence. The worker, not the work, is the focus of the testing.

A related type of testing (not addressed in this chapter) is work capacity evaluation, designed specifically for a certain job. For example, if Clarence were a welder, then he would be given a test that simulated the critical demands of welding. If Clarence were a nurse, he would be given a functional test simulating the critical demands of nursing. The advantage to this type of testing is that it simulates work more closely than a generically designed FCE. If the specific job is known and Clarence has a high degree of probability of returning only to that job, then a work capacity test would be appropriate. If Clarence does not pass the welding test, however, the information gained from that is not applicable to other jobs such as nursing. Therefore, the limitation of work capacity evaluation is that its information cannot be extrapolated to critical demands of other jobs. In addition, because of the great variety in critical demands between different jobs and even within job titles for different companies, work capacity tests almost always need to be customized to the individual. This precludes standardization of the process unless many people take the same test for their jobs.

To enhance positive aspects of both a generic FCE and a work capacity evaluation, a functional capacity evaluation can add limited components of work testing not covered in a generic standardized format. This combination may be the best of both tests but does take advanced planning.

Critical Characteristics of FCE

Definition and Description

The definition of FCE is critical in determining its purpose. The following definition is positively received by referral sources such as employers, rehabilitation consultants, and physicians.[1]

Functional: Meaningful, useful, purposeful activity that is actual work movement. Functional implies a dynamic movement with a beginning and an end which can be measured.

Capacity: Maximum ability, capability. Capacity indicates existing abilities for activities including the maximal function able to be used.

Evaluation: Systematic approach including observation, measurement, reasoning, and conclusion. Evaluation goes beyond monitoring and recording and implies an outcome statement and recommendations.

Types of Functional Testing

To test active function, the motion components should be dynamic. Dynamic tests allow two choices—psychophysical and kinesiophysical. Both use functional body activity, but they differ in several significant areas:

Psychophysical (results based on a person's mental determination of their physical limits)	Kinesiophysical (results based on a professional evaluation of movement patterns to indicate level of safeness of function)
a. The client determines his or her own performance level.	a. Professional (therapist) determines maximum performance level.
b. Effort is dependent on motivation.	b. "Level of effort" is identified by objective movement criteria.
c. Safety is often left unchecked (or inferred by putting responsibility in client's hands).	c. Safety is monitored closely by therapist.
d. Physical causes for functional limitations are not identified.	d. Physical impairment relationship to function is identified.
e. Function is subjectively determined based on the client's statement.	e. Objective methods of evaluation are used and correlated with client's statement.

The psychophysical approach is often used in functional testing done in a research mode. The research subject has no vested interest in outcome and therefore is not suspect of giving anything other than a legitimate effort. The kinesiophysical approach is used as a traditional physical medicine approach of evaluating movement with its functional and dysfunctional components.

If a subject is uninjured, aware of self body function, and motivated to perform well (but not overmotivated), psychophysical performance will likely give a good indication of ability. It fails, however, with clients in a Worker's Compensation setting who have motivation pressures. Many injured workers are fearful of reinjury or equate functional discomfort with reinjury. Some workers do not wish to appear well enough to return to work, are fearful, or are noncompliant, all of which can lead to low scores.

Problems also arise in a psychophysical approach if the client is overly motivated and performance goes beyond safe levels. This can lead to a high reinjury rate. An examiner may believe that safety is ensured because the client can "stop himself." In fact, the medical professional cannot delegate the safety of the patient to the patient himself or herself. If there are injuries or negligence suits against evaluators for causing "injury," the therapist will be at risk of a negligence charge if active safety precautions have not been taken during the testing. The client is not the professional and should not be given the responsibility of safety. Accuracy can also be a problem if only the clients rate their performance. Humans are not good predictors of their own function after they are injured. Even an athlete with excellent body awareness depends on the medical professional to determine the time and level of return to sport. The less body-aware injured worker deserves the same accuracy of functional evaluation.

The kinesiophysical approach, conversely, bases scoring on the skilled evaluator's observation of functional body movements (kinesiology) and muscles and joints that are involved in that movement. A therapist can identify dysfunction as being different from normal function and can identify actual unsafe or uncontrolled movement.

Indications of effort can be identified by thorough analysis of each functional capacity item. For example, in use of muscle groups, there are gradations of effort. Primary muscle groups (prime movers) are used for light activity. Accessory muscles are recruited with heavier activity both to stabilize and to assist the prime movers. For example, in picking up a box from a table, the biceps and finger flexors are prime movers. As the lift increases from light to moderate, accessory muscles are recruited. Not only will the biceps and finger flexor muscles begin to bulge, but there will also be a notable increase in activity in the upper trapezius. When heavy activity begins, there will be noticeable neck flexor stabilization, increased upper trapezius use, and deltoid activity. This staging of muscle function allows the therapist to note what level of activity is being used. Ongoing research studies by Isernhagen and Associates, Inc. are designed to show the reliability of these observations.

Identification of the physical problem that relates to a dysfunction relies on the kinesiophysical skill of the therapist. In gait analysis, for example, therapists can identify the difference between a gluteus medius weakness limp and one caused by ankle instability. These can be linked with muscle or joint stability testing of the hip and ankle muscles. Just as there is a difference between these two types of gait deviations, there are also differences in muscle dysfunction in functional capacity testing. Lifts that are limited by quadriceps weakness will have a different movement pattern than those that are limited by biceps weakness. Once the weaknesses are identified, the therapist can make appropriate recommendations.

Regarding safety, if a client begins to lose safe, controlled movement, the therapist should stop the test. Even a motivated client who wishes to lift heavy loads in order to go back to work will need to be stopped when safety is compromised. Return to work is not the only outcome. Only when safe functional work can be accomplished is there a positive result. If the client wishes to return to a job that requires more ability than he or she currently has, a remedial program can be suggested. Extremely high motivation should not be seen as a reason to push beyond safe limits.

Standardized Testing

Functional Capacity Testing, because it comes from a list of specific items (Figure 8.1), can be standardized. Standardization involves developing specific methods for testing all items to be included in the testing procedure. For example, there may be twenty functional capacity items ranging from lifting to forward bending to ambulation activities. Procedures should be written including purpose, functional patterns, equipment, and scoring criteria. Standardization ensures that each test item will always be administered and scored with the same approach. This avoids rater bias. Results will be directly related to the client's performance. Referral sources and clients can be confident in the procedures.

Test-retest capability exists with a standardized format. In many cases the client undergoing FCE will be retested either after return to work or after a work hardening program. If the test has not been standardized, retest information will not be valuable.

Another benefit of using a standardized test is in planning and execution. Once the therapist is well trained in administration of the test and has a thorough understanding of interpretation and recommendations, each test performed will allow greater expertise to develop.

Length of Functional Capacity Evaluation

Comprehensiveness, clarity, and test design are primary criteria for obtaining valid information from FCE. These criteria can be directly tied to intensity and length of the FCE. Time parameters include the number of total hours a test is performed and the number of days over which the test is performed.

If one is to administer a 1- or 2-hour test, it is likely that not all twenty items listed in estimated functional capacity forms will be tested. Therefore, any short test will most likely not cover all of the critical items asked on functional capacity forms. To perform adequate physical testing of all the FCE items required, the minimum amount of time required is generally 4 to 6 hours.

A second decision involves the number of days of testing. The benefit of doing testing portions on a second or third day is the ability to evaluate the effect that the test items have had on the client. The following are examples:

- A worker with a degenerative joint condition may have an exacerbation of this condition (warmth, swelling, and decrease in motion) after the joint has been stressed. Since actual work needs to be at a threshold that will not inflame the joint, the second day reevaluation is critical.
- A second day reevaluation will also allow identification of increased pain even though there is not a related increase in pathological problems or dysfunction. This type of discomfort may be related to normal muscle stress of an area that has not previously been exercised. If simple muscle soreness is noted, it is important to point out to a client that this is not a new injury but rather an indication for conditioning.
- Fearful clients may find it difficult to fully overcome their fear on the first day of testing and test better on the second day. The second day testing gives them the opportunity to establish their own self-image on work ability. The conclusion that they are "able to do more" than they thought is a positive reinforcement.

The ability to obtain consistency of results through a 2-day test will increase the reliability of FCE outcome and recommendations. Telephone follow-ups are not adequate. Only professional identification of second-day function or dysfunction can be considered objective.

Cooperation of Client

The client must work to physical capacity maximums in order for true abilities to be noted. This is important to discuss at the beginning of the test. If the client is fearful, it is helpful to note that the examiner will be watching safety criteria during the entire test. Therefore, the fearful person can leave safety in the hands of the therapist and does not need to self-limit in order to remain safe.

The therapist-client relationship is also important to establish. Therapists are nonadversarial in this return-to-work process. They will be examining the client for true abilities and limitations. The outcome biases of the client, employer, or any attorney involved are not considered.

In most cases, the therapist-client discussion of the purpose of the test, its safety, and the need for objective information encourages client cooperation. At the end of the test, results should be discussed with the client. The client should also receive a copy of the test results in writing as any return to work needs to be agreed to by the client as well as the employer and the physician.

Difficult Clients

One type of difficult client is the person who perceives that pain interferes with function. If the client allows this pain to stop functional activities, correlation needs to be made with the physical impairment. The therapist is educated in pathological problems and should also study the client's history and injury pattern. Symptoms that relate to pathological problems should be observed and documented. This shows a pathological reason for the discomfort and functional limitation. Beyond that, however, many patients have "pain behaviors" that are not wholly based on physical problems. Tests such as the Waddell signs are effective to help determine when a response is due to a nonphysiological problem.[5,6]

The decision to work "with discomfort" is the client's. Clients can begin to take control of their own activity and see if they can work through the perceived discomfort that has always stopped them in the past. It is their choice. The outcome statement will be related to whether the end of the test is due to their own self-limitation (stopping before heavy effort is identified) or to a physical cause related to the impairment. The benefit of encouraging full activity at safe levels is that true functional levels can then be determined. If a therapist does not encourage clients to perform fully, pain behavior patients may never realize their full potential.

The second category of difficult client is the one who deliberately exaggerates behavior or who attempts to fake disability. This person exhibits nonphysiological physical patterns. These might include staggering, exaggerated holding of body parts, and dramatically exhibiting signs of severe stress on areas that are not actually stressed by the test.[5,6] Such behaviors should be documented. The client should be informed that the behavior is not consistent with the test item. The therapist should remain objective and not become upset with the client. As Waddell noted, these are signs that the client needs psychological evaluation. They are not justification for giving the client a negative label. The outcome statement should reflect that the client had "exaggerated behaviors that limited him/her functionally, but were not caused by physical limitations."

Testing Format

History

The client must be comfortable in knowing the purpose of the test. In the initial interview, it is helpful to state that the test is objective and the information will relate to the person's physical ability. The examiner is not working for either the employee or the employer, and there is no vested interest in either side. The results will be used, however, to determine abilities and limitations in relationship to work.

Often, the client reporting for a functional evaluation is already in some type of discomfort. This should be documented by the examiner. If necessary, a short discussion on the difference between function and discomfort (pain) should be held.

In the history, the evaluator discusses the cause of injury with the client. It is important to determine how healing from the injury has progressed and how the client is currently affected by the physical condition. Inquiring about current exercise programs, current activities at home or in recreations, and level of functioning in daily activities is helpful in establishing a baseline. If the client has found that high levels of activity increase discomfort or symptoms, the examiner will indicate that the FCE activities might similarly increase such symptoms. The client should be encouraged to return on the second day, regardless of whether there is more discomfort present or the client feels better. As mentioned previously, the second (or third) day verifies performance levels and/or dysfunctions.

Brief Physical Exam before Testing

There are two primary reasons to perform a scanning physical assessment prior to FCE: (1) to clear the worker from physical contraindications to the test and define physical parameters that must be monitored for safety during the testing process; and (2) to provide information on impairment which can then be linked to functional limitations found in the testing. This is critical for credibility and medical-legal interpretation.

In the first instance, the therapist should seek to obtain a referral for testing from a physician. This allows any medical contraindications to be stated. These may include cardiac precautions, musculoskeletal problems not evident (i.e., fusion not yet fully healed), or other medical conditions that need to be addressed during testing. Many clients have pathological physical conditions in addition to their work injury diagnosis which are important to consider during the testing procedure.

Even with a physician referral, the therapist is not absolved from the responsibility of ensuring client safety during testing. General muscle strength, muscle imbalances, joint integrity, loss of motion or flexibility, high blood pressure or heart rate, and so on are important to discover and monitor. For example, knee instability or a significant chondromalacia might preclude heavy load lifting from the floor. Identifying these limitations helps to avoid exacerbating symptoms during the testing procedure.

If hearings or legal proceedings utilize results from a functional capacity evaluation, impairment measurements such as range of motion or muscle

ISERNHAGEN WORK SYSTEMS
FUNCTIONAL CAPACITY EVALUATION ITEMS

HISTORY	UNWEIGHTED ROTATION TOLERANCE
Musculoskeletal Physical (brief)	Sitting
LIFTS	Standing
Floor to Waist	LOW ACTIVITIES
Waist to Overhead	Crawl
Horizontal	Kneel
PUSH/PULL	Crouch
Static	Repetitive Squat
Dynamic	AMBULATION ACTIVITIES
CARRY	Walking
Front	Stair Climbing
Right Handed	Step Ladder Climbing
Left Handed	STATIC WORK
ELEVATED WORK	Sitting
FORWARD BENDING TOLERANCE	Standing
Sitting	UPPER EXTREMITY
Standing	Hand Grip
	Coordination

Figure 8.2 Isernhagen work systems functional capacity evaluation items.

strength can be linked to the functional problems. In legal proceedings it is often the examiner with the most specific objective data whose testimony is considered more accurate. The accuracy of testing depends on accurate preliminary measurements. Standards of practice will increasingly indicate that functional capacity evaluations must be preceded by a preliminary examination.[7]

Evaluation Items

An example of the Isernhagen Functional Capacity Evaluation is shown in Figure 8.2 and Table 8.1. Beyond this skeleton procedure format, the therapist must write the procedures and additional scoring criteria for each facility. Training of each therapist in FCE should be done, with competencies noted. If the procedures for evaluation, scoring, and writing reports are followed, the facility can ensure quality and consistency. In addition documented training becomes the basis for medical-legal scrutiny (Table 8.1).

Table 8.1

Evaluation Item	Objective	Movement parameters	Equipment
Lifting			
A. Floor to center of gravity (CG); vertical	Lift weight receptacle (WR) from floor to client CG	Begin at CG shelf height (adjusted to client), lower WR to floor and return; 5 repetitions	Weight receptacle approximately 12 in × 12 in × 12 in Weights Adjustable shelving
B. CG to eye level; vertical	Lift weight receptacle (WR) from CG level to eye level	Begin at CG level, raise WR to shelf height at eye level (adjusted) and return; 5 repetitions	As above
C. CG to CG; horizontal	Lift WR from CG level, move horizontally 4 ft and place at same level	Begin at CG shelf height, pivot, move 4 ft, touch WR to shelf, return; 5 repetitions	As above
Carry			
A. Bilateral front	Carry WR in two-handed manner at CG level	Begin with WR at CG level, carry 50 ft.	As above
B. Right-handed	Carry WR in one-handed manner at thigh level	Begin with WR at thigh level shelf height, carry 50 ft using right upper extremity	One-handed weight receptacle: 10 in × 12 in × 12 in with handle in middle
C. Left-handed	As above	As above; use left upper extremity	As above Maximum poundage
Push/Pull			
A. Push	Move weight sled horizontally 10 ft	Handle adjusted to chest level on weight sled, using smooth force, push 10 ft	Weight sled with adjustable push/pull bar Scale-dynamometer
B. Pull	As above	As above; pull 10 ft	As above

Handgrip

A. Right	Find maximum isometric handgrip strength	With elbow at 90 degrees use maximum grip force to squeeze handle; use 1st, 2nd, 3rd, and 4th positions	Jamar-type dynamometer Tape measure

Elevated Work

Neck/back in extension position	Work with upper extremities in elevated position while standing	Place assembly objects on shelf at worker eye level. Assemble items; 5 min. maximum	Simple assembly activity Adjustable workbench

Lowered or Forward Work

Neck/back in flexion position	Work in the position of hip and trunk flexion.		Simple assembly activity Adjustable workbench
A. Standing	• while standing	Stand with hips/trunk flexed to 20 degrees	
B. Sitting	• while sitting	Sit with hips flexed at 110 degrees	As above and stool

Unweighted Rotation

A. Standing	Move through diagonal and horizontal rotation patterns	Move through three patterns: 1. Full right to left and reverse 2. Low right to high left 3. Low left to high right; 10 cycles each	Empty, light-weight boxes, 12 in × 12 in × 12 in Adjustable shelving
B. Sitting	• while standing • while sitting		Straight-back chair without arms
Crawl	Crawl on all fours	Reciprocal crawl 30 ft	Carpeted floor
Kneel	Kneel in upright position	Knees flexed to 90 degrees Hip extended; 1 min	Carpeted floor

Table 8.1 (continued)

Sustained Crouch	Maintain full knee and hip flexion position	Position in flexed crouch; maintain 1 min	Rail for balance
Repetitive Squat	Flex hips and knees fully to touch hands to floor	Stand, squat, return to stand; maximum 1 min, minimum 10 repetitions	Rail for balance
Stair Ambulation	Ascend and descend steps	Ascend and descend a flight of stairs until 100 have been traversed	Flight of stairs
Balance and Stabilization	Step through lattice of squares while walking, demonstrating balance	Walk 40 ft with correct foot placement in squares, both diagonal and line pattern	Thin lattice of 18 in squares 10 ft long, 2 ft wide
Sitting	Sit in chair while performing table activity	Sit, weight shifting allowed, 30 min while performing hand tests	Standard armless, padded chair with straight back. Supplemental items; lumbar roll, armrests
Upper Extremity Coordination	Perform designated fine and gross motor coordination tests	Follow directions on hand coordination tests	As specified by hand coordination test
Right			
Left			

Optional Functional Capacity Evaluation Items

Walking

Running

Standing

Outdoor Activity—Uneven Terrain

Driving

Step Tests

Upper Extremity Cumulative Work

Functional Capacity Evaluation Written Report

Essentials of Report

The written report should be in clear, direct language, absent of as much medical jargon as possible. Besides the physician, the readers will be the employer, the rehabilitation consultant, the insurance company, and Worker's Compensation representatives. The reader should get a clear picture of physical capabilities and limitations as they relate to critical demands of the job. In addition, there should be clearly written job modifications and recommendations for any further intervention. After reading the written report, the reader should clearly understand how the case is best resolved. The two main components of the report are the summary letter and recommendations.

Summary Letter

The summary letter (Figure 8.3) reviews all items on the Functional Capacity Evaluation form. Included are the following topics:

I. Cooperation and consistency of the client during the testing procedure. This may include internal consistency checks such as Waddell signs.
  1. If the client demonstrated consistency of performance, this can be stated in three areas.
     a. There was consistency between like items being tested (e.g., overhead work and waist to eye level lifting).
     b. There was consistency of symptoms and physical diagnosis (e.g., bending activity, dysfunction, and spondylolisthesis).
     c. There was consistency between first- and second-day testing.
  2. If the client did not demonstrate consistency, this can be stated in nonjudgmental language, as in the following examples.
     a. In some tests stressing neck rotation, client acted guarded and would not move neck (in physical assessment and overhead work). Yet, when not aware of positioning, he moved his neck freely through a large range of motion (during hand testing and in trunk rotation test). This inconsistency shows a limitation that does not appear to be musculoskeletal.
     b. Client refused to lift any weight beyond 10 pounds in all three lifts. He was at a light effort level when he refused to go further, stating "I feel burning in my back." Therefore, he is not physically limited by strength or endurance in lifting, but is self-limited.

CASE STUDY 2
FUNCTIONAL CAPACITY EVALUATION:
SUMMARY REPORT

NAME: Hugh Van

TEST DATES: October 22 and 23, 1989

ADDRESS: 904 Clover Lane, Eugene, OR 66666

DATE OF BIRTH: 12/19/39

PHYSICIAN: Carol Henderson, MD

REFERRAL SOURCE: Anna Lauren, Occupational Health Nurse, School District #202

DIAGNOSIS: Crushing Injury, Right Upper Extremity, Fracture, Right Distal Humerus, Right Distal
Ulna,   April 16, 1989

DESCRIPTION OF TESTS DONE: Mr. Van participated in a standardized IWS Functional Capacity
Evaluation.

Cooperation: Client demonstrated cooperative behavior in that he was willing to work to his maximum
abilities throughout all test items.

Consistency of Performance: Client demonstrated a consistent performance indicated by reproducible
abilities throughout the testing procedure. There was consistency among the functional capacity items, with
the only areas of limitation being right upper extremity coordination and endurance.   There was full
consistency between the first day of testing and the second day of testing; thus, indicating that the results
gained should be valid as a basis for return to work planning.

Pain Behavior: Client demonstrated physical signs that symptoms were present during strong grasps, wrist
compression, and a repetitious fine coordination activities. There were no overt pain behaviors, however,
and the client appeared to have symptoms well in control.

Safety: The client demonstrated safe performance, including body mechanics, appropriate pacing, and
general awareness of safe techniques.

Quality of Movement: Client demonstrated smooth and coordinated movement throughout the test items,
with the exception of the right upper extremity. In this area, there was some incoordination with strong
upper extremity movements or fine hand coordination.

A

Figure 8.3 Functional capacity evaluation summary report.

    II. Safety of body movement and use of body mechanics.
   III. Major strengths regarding work activities. This delineates the abilities of the client in relation to general work categories.
   IV. Physical limitations regarding work activities. This delineates physical limitations for all work categories.
    V. Job description. This is best gained through skilled, unbiased (not client) job analysis.

Significant Abilities: Mr. Van demonstrates high abilities in lifting from the waist level, pulling left hand carry, bilateral carry, and all positional activities that include bending, sitting, standing, walking, crouching, etc. The client is not deconditioned at this point and is able to do relatively heavy work, excepting, the right upper extremity, sustained over an 8-hour day.

Significant Deficits: In regard to the right upper extremity, there has been a good functional recovery, taking into consideration the nature of the crushing injury and the fractures. There has been significant progress in strength, endurance, and coordination in the entire right upper extremity. At this point, however, the client has plateaued and continues to have mild limitations in lifting and carrying with the right upper extremity, elevated lifting or static work, ladder use or right hand grip, and coordination. The right upper extremity is functional for many gross motor activities and the use of the extremity is encouraged.

Job Descriptions Explored: The client's previous employment as the maintenance person is School District #202 is available. The duties include use of long-handled tools, such as mops, brooms, shovels, etc.; painting of surfaces with whole body reach; cleaning of areas using upper extremities with whole body reach; and general inspection of school areas.

Physical Work Strengths Compared to Job Description: Client will be able to use long-handled tools well, as long as he can take frequent changes of activity when the right upper extremity becomes fatigued. He will be able to carry and lift all pails, boxes, etc., required on the job, as long as they are not lifted above shoulder level. Client has capability for standing, walking, bending, squatting, and other positions required for the job. He also appears to have endurance in aerobic capacity which will sustain this activity over an 8-hour day.

Physical Restrictions Compared to Job Description: The client will not be able to lift heavy objects above shoulder level due to right upper extremity decreased strength and lack of tolerance to compression. Overhead work, such as painting and cleaning, will also have to be limited for the right upper extremity. This should be able to be done primarily with the left upper extremity or modified with the use of other tools. In addition, fine hand activities, such as use of a screwdriver, pins, nails, etc., may be difficult for the client. The left hand can be used and the right hand can be used for hand coordination activities, however.

Recommendations:

1. Physical abilities do match the job description of maintenance person for the school district. The only areas of discrepancy will be in the right upper extremity, fine motor coordination, and in heavy overhead work. Ladders may also be a problem if he is required to carry equipment. Overall, however, the client has the physical abilities to return to work with the modifications indicated in this report.

2. One modification at work that will be helpful would be the changing of shelving in the storeroom to accommodate more low shelves and no shelves over shoulder height. As the client progresses in strength with work and exercise program, however, this may be able to be increased.

3. Physical therapy for four more weeks tapering to home program to continue progress in the right upper extremity and to increase mobility and strength of all areas. This will not interfere with immediate return to work, however, as appointments can be made outside work hours.

B

Figure 8.3 (continued)

Recommendations

After the functional capacity evaluation form and letter are completed, the therapist will make recommendations based on the objective evidence. In all cases the recommendations will be maintained within the professional scope of practice. The following are potential recommendations.

1. "Physical capabilities of the worker match the critical demands of the job, thus indicating the physical ability to return to work," or

"physical abilities of the client do not match the critical demands of the job, therefore necessitating. . . ."

2. If there is not a clear match between critical demands and functional abilities, the following recommendations can be made:
   • Modification of the work to reduce poundage, change positions, use job rotation, use adaptive equipment, and so on.
   • Modification of the client by referral to physical therapy, occupational therapy, or a rehabilitation program directed at return to work that would involve work conditioning or work hardening.
3. Referral back to the physician or to another practitioner for further evaluation. This may happen if there are physical problems that have been previously undiagnosed or that require further medical evaluation. In addition, there may be other concerns such as psychological or emotional overlay, nutritional problems, or potential chemical dependency which were noted during the testing. These should be referred to the appropriate professionals.

The recommendations will allow movement toward case resolution. All recommendations should be substantiated by objective evidence found in the FCE report. Recommendations are the therapist's final statement in regard to potential case resolution.

Functional Capacity Evaluation Form

As noted at the beginning of this chapter, a form such as the Estimated Functional Capacity Form (Figure 8.4) should be completed. This is a standard release to work. This is the therapist's form and does not constitute a medical release to work as this coordinates with the role of the physician. If the physician chooses to use it as a release, he or she will sign the FCE form which then becomes part of the return-to-work information. It should accompany all written Functional Capacity Evaluation results.

Functional Capacity Evaluation Report Dissemination

The Functional Capacity Evaluation report is important in all aspects of return to work. All of the team members involved in the client's return to work should receive a copy of the report. Going into the test the client should be aware that a report will be sent to all interested parties. Also, conferences may be scheduled after the FCE so that all interested parties in the return-to-work process or case resolution discuss the results of the FCE.

Hugh Van
Client

October 22 and 23, 1989
Date

Item	Percent of 8-hour Day					Restrictions	Recommendations
	0	1-5	6-33	34-66	67-100		
WEIGHT CAPACITY IN LBS.							
Floor to waist lift		55	40	30	20	Decreased r. elbow, wrist, and hand strength	
Waist to overhead lift		15	5	0	0	Inability to tolerate deviation/ compression r. wrist	Limit overhead lifting as much as possible
Horizontal lift		95	60	30	20		
Push		40	20	5	5	Inability to tolerate compression r. wrist & elbow	Push primarily with left arm
Pull		110	80	50	30		
Right carry		20	15	10	5	Decreased r. elbow wrist, and hand strength	
Left carry		55	40	30	15		
Front carry		95	60	30	20		
Right hand grip		70	40	20	5	Decreased strength of flexors	
Left hand grip		120	90	60	40		
FLEXIBILITY/POSITIONAL							
Elevated work			X			Low endurance, right arm	Frequent rest breaks
Forward bending/sitting					X		
Forward bending/standing					X		

Figure 8.4 Estimated functional capacity form.

Recipients of Report

The following people should receive FCE reports:

1. *Physical therapist and occupational therapist:* for treatment and evaluation.
2. *Physician:* to authorize return to work or direct further medical management.
3. *Rehabilitation counselors/vocational consultants:* to facilitate the return-to-work process by working with medical providers, the employer, and the insurance company.
4. *Insurance companies and Worker's Compensation systems:* for case resolution.
5. *Employers:* for placement of the worker at work.
6. *Attorneys:* for case resolution.
7. *The worker:* The most important person is the worker. The FCE has specific information relating to the individual's own work and life. The worker is the person who most needs to be aware of safe work function and also to be able to limit unsafe work functions. To promote productivity and safety, the worker must be fully aware of his or her own physical parameters.

Conference

An FCE conference allows results to be explained to all parties interested in the client's return to work. At this conference specific questions that go beyond the scope of the report may be asked. A return-to-work plan is often begun at this point. Benefits of the conference are that the worker hears the full report and the employer can make plans for the worker's return to work. Any of the medical, vocational, or rehabilitation professionals involved will be merely facilitory to that process.

Future Perspectives

Blending Science with Art

Because of the need for impairment and disability information, greater emphasis on actual functioning of the body with appropriate references to physical impairment will be necessary. Physical abilities regarding work must be acceptable to the employer, employee, and all parties in the Worker's Compensation system. When objective evidence based on the strength, weaknesses, and motions of the body are reported, all concerned will have confidence in the outcome.

Is there functional quantification by technology? Currently, there is no technology that accurately measures functional capacities such as carrying, bending, stooping, sitting, standing, climbing, and very rarely lifting. Because reliability in technology is predicated on measuring relatively few variables, it cannot have the broad scope of a comprehensive, wholistic functional capacity evaluation. Technology can, however, measure portions of body movement not seen by the human eye and will play an important part in verifying the impairment portion of the functional capacity evaluation. Technological advances in equipment now allow us to measure specific components. Examples are lumbar motion monitors, strength testing devices (dynamic), motion analyzers, and so on.

The future blending of FCE and technological measurement will be in the use of technology to *verify* what the therapist can observe in a wholistic evaluation. Technology, however, will not replace the therapist who is able to look at multitudes of variables at once including safe, controlled movement patterns. Technology and professional human evaluation will continue to interact. The gold standard will continue to be performance with actual weights and movement patterns, rather than those simulated by technology.

Medical-Legal Implications

Functional Capacity Evaluations are used increasingly in Worker's Compensation hearings and in legal cases to determine ability versus disability in settlements. This brings scrutiny of test standardization and qualifications of the evaluator. Issues brought out in medical-legal hearings include:

1. The credibility of the examiner. This takes into account professional background such as formal education in physical therapy or occupational therapy, training in being a functional capacity evaluator, and the background of the therapist in evaluating injured workers or those with physical disabilities that affect work.

2. The testing method. The objectivity and scientific manner in which a FCE is carried out are scrutinized by attorneys. If the therapist relies on the client's subjective opinion to determine maximum effort, this does very little to enhance the credibility of the therapist. Specific, objective observations and data are needed. The therapist as an expert witness is called on to use his or her background in showing how the client was evaluated. This background concerns both pathological conditions and the kinesiological approach.

3. The therapist or functional capacity evaluator is also subject to the charge of negligence when performing FCEs. For that reason, policies and procedures of testing must be documented. Client safety is an issue in these

suits, and the amount of documentation regarding client safety in test performance is important in defense against negligence suits.

4. Written policies and procedures addressing each test item, how it is to be performed, scoring criteria, and safety of procedures can protect the therapist in the event of a negligence suit.

Medical-legal credibility must be compatible with the development of more efficient, objective, clear, and safer FCEs. The tendency to remain non-adversarial will become even more important as legal proceedings occur. A good FCE is a statement of objective documentation and could readily be used by either side or both sides in hearings. The client and the employer must know that the information gained in a FCE is of a nonadversarial nature because it is objective medical testing.

Functional Capacity Evaluation Is Part of the Work Injury Management Spectrum

Functional Capacity Evaluation has been used in the past as a return-to-work evaluation. That use has been very effective in defining when a worker has the critical functional abilities to match the critical demands of the job. FCE, when performed in a timely manner, can facilitate safe, early return to work.

Traditionally, FCE has been used after a person's case has become "chronic" or "difficult." In such cases, the FCE has proven valuable by clearly defining disabilities that lead to referral into a work conditioning or work hardening program. The rehabilitation program then allows increases in function and work ability. At the end of the program, part of the discharge evaluation will be another FCE, putting into formal terms the outcome abilities and limitations. These then are matched with job demands so the client can return to work.

As employers become more familiar with work modification and as medical professionals adopt the philosophy of early return to work, functional evaluation can become abbreviated in order to be used much earlier in the spectrum. The therapist can perform a valuable service by completing a functional evaluation with moderately injured individuals at the end of acute treatment, in the early weeks after injury. This places the worker back at work at a productive, yet safe, level sooner. This may help avoid the "light duty/nonproductive" pool where the person is physically at work, but not actually productive.

The third area of progress for functional evaluation will be in prework screening. With the passage of the Americans with Disabilities Act,[8] there now is a need to limit medical screening in two ways. First, medical screening is limited to companies and situations that can show it is necessary for business. To prevent discrimination, the employer must also demonstrate that the screening is functionally related to the job demands.

By developing functional job descriptions and identifying critical demands, prework screening will then be done, when necessary, by evaluating a person in conjunction with the critical physical demands of the job. According to the guidelines of the Americans with Disabilities Act, the following will be necessary:

1. Medical screening will take place only after a job has been offered to an applicant;
2. All persons applying for that particular position will be screened;
3. Screening information will be kept in separate files; and
4. The medical screening must be specifically related to the job.

In summary, Functional Capacity Evaluation has not only found its niche with the difficult client, but it can also be used effectively in the early return-to-work process and even before injury happens. Its use ensures placement of a worker in employment that matches his or her functional ability.

Further Expansion of FCE

Functional Capacity Evaluation will become increasingly important as safe work continues to be emphasized, both for injured and uninjured workers. For example, the Commission on Accreditation of Rehabilitation Facilities (CARF) has promulgated accreditation criteria for work hardening programs. One of the features of this accreditation is that no client will enter a work hardening program without a thorough evaluation of the program's feasibility. It is possible that the FCE described in this chapter could meet three or four test types, especially with functional work matching the job title categories.

Taking an active stand, unions and employers will become more proactive in insisting on better match of an injured worker to the job. This is important for prevention of reinjury and also for entering the worker at the highest productivity level. An FCE that is objective and accurate in defining physical capacities is nonadversarial and will benefit both labor and management. The Americans with Disabilities Act, which was previously discussed in regard to functional capacity screening, also states the need for employers to make reasonable work accommodations for injured or handicapped employees. A thorough FCE with modification recommendations will enhance the employers' ability to do this.

Summary

Throughout this chapter the practical application of functional evaluation has been explored. Worker's Compensation, unions, management, and disabled workers benefit from results of worker/work matching. Two issues, however, still loom on the horizon as practical questions. How can one find quality providers of FCE, and how will this quality evaluation be funded? Scrutiny of accuracy and usefulness to insurance companies may ultimately be the bottom line.

Accreditation agencies, Worker's Compensation systems, new legislation, and employers will continue to increase use of functional assessments as long as their needs are being met. Outcomes studies of worker/work matching will have to show progress in both the financial and human work experience arenas of industry. Comprehensive functional capacity evaluation reimbursement will be on quality, rather than on price. The future of functional capacity evaluation, therefore, is driven by science, medical-legal implications, and reimbursement issues. If it can accommodate and work with these pressures, FCE not only will remain an important factor in the injured worker spectrum, but also will continue to improve in scope, accuracy, and usefulness. It is a cornerstone of matching the worker and the work.

References

1. Isernhagen S: Functional capacity evaluation. In Isernhagen S. (ed) Work Injury: Management and Prevention. Rockville, MD. Aspen Publishers, 1988.
2. Isernhagen S: The role of functional capacity assessment after rehabilitation. In Bullock M. (ed) Ergonomics: The Physiotherapist in the Workplace. London, Churchill-Livingstone, 1990.
3. Key G: Work capacity analysis. In Scully R., Barnes M (ed). Physical Therapy. Philadelphia, Lippincott, 1989.
4. Miller M: Functional assessments. Work 1:3, 1991.
5. Waddell G, McCulloch J, Kummel E, et al: Nonorganic physical signs in low back pain. Spine 5:2, 1980.
6. Waddell G, Main C, Morris E, et al: Chronic low back pain, psychologic distress, and illness behavior. Spine 9:2, 1984.
7. Hart D, Matheson L, Isernhagen S: Task Force Report on Tests and Measurements. ERRS, Duluth, MN, 1992
8. The Americans with Disabilities Act. The Bureau of National Affairs, Inc. Washington, D.C., 1990.

9

□ □ □
□ □ □
□ □ □
□ □ □

Objective
Quantification of
Trunk Performance

Mohamad Parnianpour
Jackson C. Tan

Editor's Note: Trunk dynamometry is rapidly emerging as an important clinical tool for examining many facets of LBP. At this time, research is advancing but still limited. This chapter defines those limitations by critically assessing both completed and ongoing research. The reader should be impressed by the complexity of this process and thereby made more cautious about clinical interpretation without more specific information on protocols and outcome measures.

Research on trunk dynamometers has yet to demonstrate that underlying pathology or even specific patho-mechanics can be accurately evaluated from trunk dynamometry data. They are appropriately used only as a measuring tool to guide clinicians in decision making. The assumption that pathology can be identified by a dynamometer is not new. Chondromalacia patellae was one such pathological entity that was thought to be observable with isokinetic knee dynamometry. As this has proven to be false, the clinician should be cautious about interpreting even more complex information from a trunk dynamometer.

An even greater potential for abuse with trunk dynamometry remains in the field of litigation. Trunk dynamometers have been promoted as being able to identify patients who are malingering. As this chapter demonstrates, the complexities of data generated from trunk dynamometers make such sweeping generalizations regarding the sincerity of a patient's test improbable. The enigma of this information is that while the data generated are objective, psychosocial variables such as fear, anxiety, and depression are known to influence a patient's motivation.

While the sophistication of engineering concepts in trunk dynamometry can seem tedious to a clinician, this information is vital for interpreting data from trunk dynamometers. When combined with the case studies in Chapter 10, the specific application of trunk dynamometry to clinical care provides the reader with an exciting new tool to aid in the rehabilitation process.

The inability to correlate low back pain (LBP) to anatomical findings and the difficulties in quantifying pain have directed much effort toward quantification of performance of spinal function. Assessment of function across various dimensions of performance (such as strength, endurance, and coordination) has provided the basis for a rational approach to clinical assessment, rehabilitation strategies, and determination of return to work potential for injured employees. To understand the complex problem of LBP, terminologies related to trunk muscle exertion and performance must first be defined.

Muscle Exertion and Performance

The four fundamental types of muscle exertion or action are isometric, isokinetic, isotonic, and isoinertial. In *isometric* exertion, muscle length is constant and there is no joint movement. Although mechanical work is not achieved, physiological work, that is, static work, is performed and energy is consumed.[1,2] When the internal force exerted by the muscle is greater than the external force offered by the resistance, then concentric or shortening muscle action occurs; whereas if the muscle is already activated and the external force offered by the resistance exceeds the internal force of the muscle, then eccentric or lengthening muscle action occurs.[3,4]

When the muscle moves, either concentrically or eccentrically, dynamic work is performed.[2] If the joint velocity or rate of shortening or lengthening of the muscle is constant, the exertion is called *isokinetic.*[5,6] When the muscle acts on a constant inertial mass, the exertion is called *isoinertial.*[7] *Isotonic* exertion occurs when the muscle tension is constant throughout the range of motion.[6] Isotonic exertion, as defined, is not realizable physiologically because muscular tensions change as the lever arms of the joint change, despite the constancy of external loads.[6]

These terminologies as employed in the literature are imprecise and confusing. While the terms are intended to refer to the state of muscles, they actually refer to the state of the mechanical interface, that is, the dynamometer. Because muscles usually shorten or lengthen at varying rates and tensions, it is clear that isokinetic and isoinertial movements are somewhat artificial and are usually produced by constraining a subject to a device such as a dynamometer, which helps to control limb segment speed, range of motion, and/or resistance.[8] During isometric action, the effect of the generated tension is less than the external resistance, thus, the external load does not displace. Muscle length will remain constant only if the joint posture is "controlled" by the use of soft constraints (verbal instruction) or hard constraints (stabilization straps).

For any joint or joint complex, muscle performance can be quantified in terms of the basic dimensions of performance: strength, speed, endurance, steadiness, and coordination. Muscle strength is the capacity to produce torque or work by voluntary activation of the muscles. Muscle endurance is the ability to maintain a predetermined level of motor output (e.g., torque, velocity, range of motion, work, or energy) over a period of time.[7] Smidt et al. defined muscle strength as the ability of a muscle or muscle group to generate a moment about a body axis; muscle endurance is the ability to generate moments repetitively.[9] Fatigue is considered to be a process under which the capability of muscles diminishes. However, neuromuscular adjustments take place to meet the task demands (i.e., increase in neural excitation) until there is final performance breakdown—endurance time. Coordination, in this context, is the temporal and spatial organization of movement and the recruitment patterns of the muscle synergies.

Despite proliferation of various technologies for measurement, basic questions such as what needs to be measured and how it can best be measured remain unanswered. Strength is one of the most fundamental dimensions of human performance and has been the focus of many investigations. There is general consensus about the abstract definition of strength: the ability to generate tension in a muscle. However, since there is no direct method for measurement of muscle tension *in vivo*, strength has often been measured at the interface of a joint (or joints) with the mechanical environment. A dynamometer, which is an external apparatus onto which the body exerts force or torque, is used to measure strength indirectly.[10]

From a physiological point of view, the measured force or torque applied at the interface is a function of: (1) the individual's motivation (magnitude of the neural drive for excitation and activation processes); (2) environmental conditions (muscle length, rate of change of muscle length, nature of the external load, metabolic conditions, pH level, temperature, and so forth); (3) prior history of activation (fatigue); (4) instruction and descriptions of the tasks given to the subject; (5) the control strategies and motor programs employed to satisfy the demands of the task; and (6) the biophysical state of the muscles and fitness (fiber composition, physiological cross-sectional area of the muscle, cardiovascular capability). It cannot be overemphasized that these processes are complex and interrelated.[4]

Different modes of strength testing have evolved based on varying technological sophistication. The mechanical conditions within the body, for example, lever arm of the tendon attachment, is difficult to quantify accurately but can be estimated by using data on cadaver studies, or by using computerized axial tomography scan (CAT scan) or magnetic resonance imaging (MRI) techniques on live human beings. The practical implication of contextual dependencies of the strength measures on the provided mechanical environment is often neglected.

To classify the various methods of strength measurements, it is necessary to identify the dependent, independent, controlled, and confounding variables. The independent variables are purposefully manipulated, while the dependent variables are quantified to show the effects of such manipulation. Controlled variables are carefully maintained at preestablished conditions to minimize their interference on the relationship of dependent and independent variables. Uncontrolled variables that may interfere with the aforementioned relationship are called *confounding* variables.[4] Kroemer et al. present concrete examples and classify variables for prevailing modes of strength testing as well as for some that are not yet utilized (e.g., isojerk).[4]

For the remainder of this chapter, static and dynamic trunk strength measurement techniques are discussed. The theoretical and practical consequences of uniaxial and triaxial dynamometers are presented.

Static (Isometric) Trunk Strength Measurements

Static strength has been measured in terms of either the force applied to the thoracic constraint or the torques generated about the axis of the dynamometer. Dynamometers used to measure isometric strength of the trunk muscles include cable tensiometers, strain-gauge dynamometers, and dynamometers used primarily for dynamic testings.

Cable Tensiometers

Cable tensiometers consist of a harness connected to a cable which is attached to a fixed object such as a wall or floor.[11] When the harness, which is strapped around the individual's chest, is pulled, the cable is stretched. The tension in the cable is then measured in calibrated units on a tension-sensitive gauge. This device was popularized by Clarke who reported an intertester reliability of 0.90 for trunk flexion and 0.99 for trunk extension.[12] Alston et al.[13] and Nachemson and Lindh,[14] using the cable tensiometer, demonstrated weakness of the trunk extensor and abdominal muscles in patients with low back pain. The disadvantage of the cable tensiometer is that it neglects to measure the lever arm distance from the center of trunk motion.[15] Also, cable tensiometers are best used to determine peak isometric torques rather than the stable average torque exerted over a 3-second period, as recommended by Caldwell et al.[16,17]

Strain-Gauge Dynamometers

Strain gauges use electroconductive materials that are sensitive to loads, that is, tension, compression, or shear.[11] When the individual pushes or pulls against the dynamometer, the gauge is deformed, leading to a change in its electrical resistance and alteration of the current passing through the gauge. The change in voltage can then be calibrated and converted into torque.

Asmussen, Heeboll-Nielsen, and Molbech (1959), cited by Mayhew and Rothstein, reported that the strain-gauge dynamometer has a reliability coefficient of 0.91 for trunk flexion and 0.92 for trunk extension.[11] Troup and Chapman used similar techniques to measure the strength of trunk extensor and abdominal muscles in healthy participants.[18] Addison and Schultz[19] and McNeill et al.[20] found that in patients with low back disorders, the trunk extensor and abdominal muscles were weaker than in healthy participants. Other investigators who used the strain-gauge dynamometer for measuring isometric trunk strength include Nicolaisen and Jorgensen;[21] Jorgensen;[22] and Kondraske et al.[23]

Dynamometers Used Primarily for Dynamic Testings

Dynamometers used for testing dynamic muscle performances contain either hydraulic or servomotor systems to provide constant velocity (e.g., isokinetic devices) or constant resistance (e.g., isoinertial devices). These dynamic devices can be locked—mechanically, through computer control, or both—for isometric strength testing. For the isometric mode of testing, most dynamic devices use strain-gauge technology, for example, the Isostation B-200 Dynamometer (Isotechnologies, Inc., P.O. Box 1239, Hillsborough, NC 27278).

Cybex isokinetic dynamometers (Cybex Division of Lumex, Inc., 2100 Smithtown Ave., Ronkonkoma, NY 11779) are the most widely used system because they were the first to be developed and made commercially available. Cybex dynamometers, which were originally used for the extremities, were adapted by several researchers for measurement of isometric trunk strength.[9,15,24-29]

The Cybex isokinetic trunk extension-flexion dynamometer, which became available commercially in 1984, was introduced in 1982 by Davies and Gould.[30] Other investigators have used this dynamometer for both isometric and isokinetic strength testing of the trunk.[30-36] Using Cybex dynamometers, the isometric strength of trunk extensor and abdominal muscles was shown to be weaker in low back pain patients compared to healthy individuals.[9,15,33]

Graves et al. used the MedX Lumbar Extension Machine (MedX Corporation, 1155 N.E. 77th St., Ocala, FL 32670), a computer-monitored dynamometer designed for testing trunk isometric strength in sitting.[37] They reported that isometric strength increased as the trunk was flexed from 0° to 72°, with an increment of 12° and that isometric training of the trunk using the device improved isometric trunk strength significantly.

Uniaxial versus Triaxial Dynamometers

Most of the existing dynamometers are uniaxial and can measure only in one plane of exertion at a time. The Lidoback (Loredan Biomedical, 1632 Da Vinci Ct., Davis, CA 95616) tests only in the sagittal plane. Cybex has two separate units for testing flexion/extension and trunk rotation. The Isostation B-200, which is the only triaxial dynamometer available commercially, is capable of measuring torque in the three planes of exertion simultaneously. There is no need to change the position of the participant when using a triaxial dynamometer as there is with the uniaxial ones, thus testing time is reduced.

Triaxial measurements are important because trunk exertions are highly coupled due to overlapping anatomical arrangements of the trunk muscles.[38-45] The primary torque dominates for most muscles as expected, that is, flexion moment for rectus abdominus and extension for longissimus dorsi. However, the accessory torques are also very important. For example, a unilateral recruitment of latissimus dorsi per unit tension (1 N) generates 30.3 (Nmm) axial torque, 45.2 (Nmm) extension torque and 42.2 (Nmm) lateral bending torque about the L3–L4 disc.[45] Each unit of tension in trunk muscles causes moments in at least two cardinal planes since they pass eccentric to the center of rotation of the motion segments.

Parnianpour et al., using a triaxial dynamometer, showed that trunk torques are coupled in all planes.[38] Studies on healthy male volunteers have shown that trunk motions occur in more than one plane. The triaxial torques and the myoelectrical activities of ten selected trunk muscles during a maximal axial rotation are shown in Figure 9.1. Buchalter et al. used a three-dimensional low-frequency magnetic field tracking device to measure the degrees of accessory motions in unrestrained trunk extension.[46] They showed that trunk motion was coupled and that triaxial coupling was less organized. It was observed that axial rotation and lateral bending are more strongly coupled due to the existing curvature of the spine in the sagittal

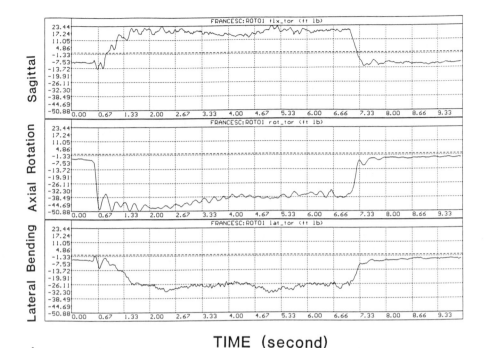

TIME (second)

A

Figure 9.1 (A) The generated triaxial torque during maximal left axial exertion and (B) the processed EMG activities (RMS = EMG) of ten selected trunk muscles during maximal trunk axial rotation in upright standing. The surface electrodes were placed at the level of the L-3 with the exception of the latissimus dorsi muscles at the T-12 level. The horizontal axis is time, in seconds. (LOB/ROB, left/right abdominal oblique; LRA/RRA, left/right rectus abdominus; LLE/RLE, left/right lateral erector spinae; LME/RME, left/right medial erector spinae; LLD/RLD, left/right latissimus dorsi.)

plane. Pearcy, Portek, and Shepherd, using three-dimensional x-ray analysis to measure intervertebral movements, also showed coupling of trunk motion in normal individuals and in patients with LBP.[47,48]

The effect of posture on coupling of the spine was first described by Lovett (1905), cited in Panjabi et al.[49] Whether increased coupling patterns indicate abnormalities in the spinal column passive structures or are caused by neuromuscular dysfunctions, or both, is still being debated. In an experiment using cadavers, Panjabi et al. studied the coupling patterns of the spinal column without the muscles. They found that posture of the spinal column (without its muscles) affects the magnitude and pattern of both the primary and coupled motions.[49] Because muscles were not studied, the effects of trunk muscle actions on coupling of movements remain unknown.

212   FUNCTIONAL CONSIDERATIONS

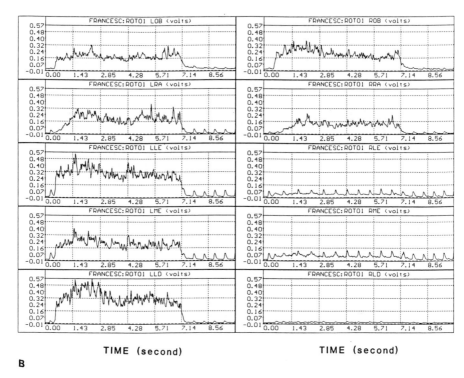

B

Figure 9.1 (continued)

Tan measured the EMG and triaxial torques of the trunk muscles to study the effect of sagittal-standing trunk posture on the coupling phenomena of the spine during isometric trunk extension in 31 healthy males.[50] Isometric trunk extension was performed with all three axes of motion locked mechanically. Accessory torques were recorded at all postures and at all exertion levels. The maximum extension torque capacity increased significantly during isometric trunk extension at 15° and 35° of trunk-flexion postures compared to 0° upright position, but the accessory torques in the transverse and coronal planes were not affected by trunk postures. The recorded lateral bending and rotation accessory torques were less than 5% and 16% of the primary extension torque, respectively.

Parnianpour et al. tested 15 male volunteers using a similar design, and reported the same results.[51] This is probably because, within the limitations of their experimental design testing healthy subjects, isometric trunk extensions were relatively pure, that is, uncoupled, and symmetrical. The effect of posture (0°, 20°, 36° of trunk flexion) significantly affected flexion and extension strength, while strength in lateral bending and axial rotation was not affected by posture. Trunk muscles were stronger at more flexed positions.[51] Accessory torque in the transverse plane was significantly increased during lateral bending exertion. This result should be viewed cautiously, since the axial torque measured by the Isostation B-200 is affected by the lateral bending torque at postures other than the upright position. Clinicians should note that only in the upright position are the axial measurements (torque and motion) valid. The mathematical correction to compensate for the crosstalk between axial rotation and lateral bending should be considered. This crosstalk, that is, influence of lateral bending on the axial rotation signals, is a result of the gimbals system design and the arrangement of the chest restraint.[51]

If future studies show significant differences in trunk coupling patterns of normal subjects and patients with low back pain, then the amount of coupling during trunk exertions could be used as an indicator of low back functional abnormality. Pearcy et al. showed that in LBP patients without nerve tension signs there is increased coupling of the spine during flexion-extension movements, indicating asymmetrical muscle action.[48]

Maximal versus Submaximal Isometric Testings

Maximal strength testing of the trunk has been used to estimate the risk of developing musculoskeletal injuries in work situations.[52,53] However, the recorded "maximum" voluntary exertion (MVE) may not always be the maximum voluntary capacity because MVE is affected by the individual's motivation and the testing circumstances.[54,55] This is especially true in complex joints, such as the trunk, where more than one muscle acts to generate the torque. To produce a truly maximum effort, all muscles, including the synergists, must simultaneously exert maximum force.[55] Because both psychological and physical factors are involved, strength measurement is considered a psychophysical technique.[56]

Biomechanical models of the trunk are usually based on static maximal strength measurement lasting for 10 to 15 seconds.[57,58] This may be misleading because in real-life work situations individuals rarely exert lengthy or maximum static effort. In fact, the recommended maximum weight for lifting should not exceed 40% to 50% of MVE of the trunk.[59] In most clinical situations, submaximal protocols are recommended, especially in patients with pain or with cardiovascular problems. Also, submaximal testings are less susceptible to fatigue and injury.[55]

Dynamic Trunk Strength Measurements

Dynamometers used to measure dynamic strength of the trunk muscle include isokinetic (Cybex Flexion/Extension Rehabilitation Unit, Cybex Torso Rotation Rehabilitation Unit, Lidoback, Kincom) and isoiner-

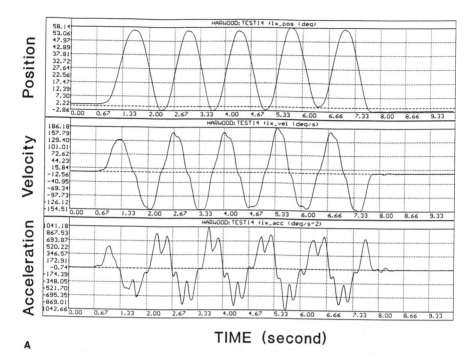

A

TIME (second)

Figure 9.2 (A) The sagittal movement profile and (B) the recruitment patterns of selected muscle activities during repetitive trunk flexion/extension in the upright position. Due to sagittal symmetry of the movement, only the right muscles are depicted. Muscles with nonsagittal orientation, obliques and latissimus dorsi muscles, do not give distinct silent period in contrast to muscles with primary sagittal orientation, the erector spinae and rectus abdominus muscles. This may be due to their contribution to the coronal stability of spine.[66] The horizontal axis is time, in seconds.

tial dynamometers (Isostation B-200). During isokinetic activity of such complex joints as the spine, only the linkage of the dynamometer has a constant angular velocity. Since the axis of rotation of the joint is not always aligned with the dynamometer and lever arms of the muscles change throughout the range of motion, no definitive statement can be made about the rate of change of muscle(s) length. General manual material handling tasks require a coordinated multilink activity which can be simulated using classical psychophysical techniques or the robotics-based lift task simulators. It has been suggested that dynamic lift simulation is close to the actual requirements of lifting tasks encountered in the industries.[60–62]

Bryant et al. determined the dynamic factors involved during an isoinertial lifting task using principal component analysis.[63] The four emerging factors emphasized the contribution of lifting technique in explaining variance

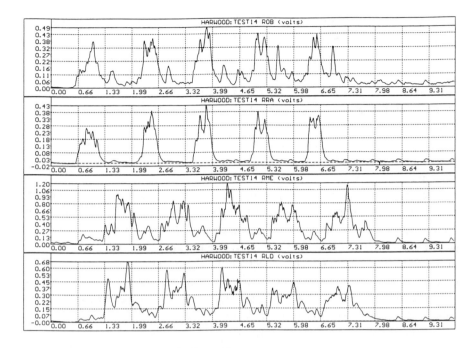

TIME (second)

B

Figure 9.2 (continued)

in isoinertial lifting strength capability. At present, the only commercially available trunk dynamometer with both isoinertial and triaxial functions is the Isostation B-200 Dynamometer. The resistance of the B-200 in each plane is set independently and the trunk is allowed to accelerate and decelerate.

Repetitive sagittal flexion/extension of the spine in the upright position and the myoelectric activities of selected trunk muscles are depicted in Figure 9.2. The phasic patterns of the extensors and flexors are markedly different from the EMG activities during isokinetic exertions. The temporal and spatial organization of recruitment and movement patterns point to a much richer and more complex media for study of low back pain. A series of theses were devoted to quantification of trunk recruitment and motor output under various mechanical conditions and types of movement.[50,64–66] Discussion of these results is beyond the scope of this chapter. The central nervous system recruits muscles with full exploitation of the gravitational field and utilizes the external resistances both for deceleration and for stabilization of the spine.[66,67] Better understanding of normal movement planning and execution may contribute to clinical care and management of LBP patients.

The commonly used B-200 protocol is the OOC (Occupational and Orthopedic Center) protocol developed by Deutsch et al.[68] This protocol is made up of the unresisted range of motion, maximum isometric exertion, and dynamic maximum performances against resistances set at 25% and 50% MVE (maximum voluntary exertion) in the three cardinal places. The tests are repeated once in reverse order of the set resistances. Performances are evaluated for a set of parameters, then compared with the previously established normal population database. The set of parameters include resisted and unresisted range of motion, maximum and average isometric and dynamic torques and velocities, and their normalized ratios (that is, max torque/resistance). The normal range of values was determined as the mean with ± 2 standard deviations.

As demonstrated by Parnianpour et al.,[69] the procedure used by Deutsch et al.[68] is only valid during measurements of one variable or an uncorrelated (independent) set of variables. To illustrate this, the performance of two subjects in the sagittal plane were compared. Subject A (Figure 9.3a & b) had a maximum isometric extension of 282.8 Nm which was ranked above the 76th percentile. His maximum velocity of 159.1 deg/sec against 50% MVE was only ranked above the 38th percentile. The maximum isometric extension of subject B (Figure 9.3c & d) was 158.9 Nm which was ranked below the 5th percentile. However, the maximum velocity obtained by subject B against 50% MVE resistance was 149.6 deg/sec which was ranked above the 34th percentile. The higher the isometric strength of a subject, the higher the absolute value of resistance will be for the same relative resistance (set resistance normalized by the MVE). Therefore, due to the inverse relation between the torque and the velocity, the stronger person may have a lower velocity (which is reflected in the covariance matrix). Based on a univariate normal distribution analysis, the strongest subjects will be assigned correctly to the top percentage of the population for their isometric measurement and will be erroneously assigned to a lower percentile based on dynamic performance parameters.

Parnianpour et al.[69] argued that the procedure used by Deutsch et al.[68] is valid only during measurements of one variable or an uncorrelated (independent) set of variables. However, the use of multivariate normal distributions requires not only the mean and variance of each variable but also the covariance matrix. The diagonal elements of the covariance matrix are the variances of the variables and the off-diagonal elements are the covariances. Therefore, the proper adjustments on torque based on its relationship (covariance) with velocity would be possible. This method is recommended when the measured variables are correlated, as is the case in isoinertial performances. This would allow for a correct ranking not only in the isometric, but in the dynamic performance as well, which may be of clinical relevance, especially in rehabilitation.

Parnianpour et al. investigated the effect of fatiguing repetitive trunk flexion and extension on movement patterns and motor output using a triaxial dynamometer.[38] The sagittal resistance was set to 70% of MVE in the

OOC Evaluation Results for **Subject A**   #112334
21-MAY-90

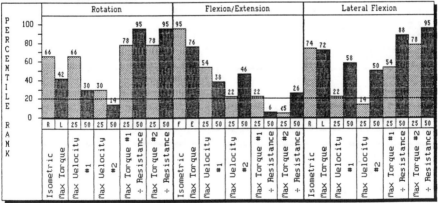

Figure 9.3 The reports of OOC protocol for two subjects. Subject A (A & B) has higher isometric strength than subject B (C & D). However, by not taking into account the absolute set resistances, the dynamic performances are erroneously scored.

OOC Evaluation Results for **Subject A**

#112334
21-MAY-90

OOC Test	Rotation	Flex/Ext	Lat Flex

Range of Motion

		Rotation	Flex/Ext	Lat Flex
ROM (deg)	#1	93.4	106.7	76.2
	#2	94.1	107.7	72.6
$\frac{ROM \#2}{ROM \#1}$ (Δ%)		0.75	0.94	-4.72↓

Isometric

	Rotation	Flex/Ext		Lat Flex
Max Torque (lb-ft)	86.0	215.6↑	208.6	148.5✕

Dynamic

		25%	50%	25%	50%	25%	50%
$\frac{Avg\ Torque}{Resistance}$ (%)	#1	112.27↑	127.44↑	101.92	101.06	96.49	96.35
	#2	115.45↑	127.44↑	101.73	100.48	99.19	96.51
$\frac{Max\ Torque}{Resistance}$ (%)	#1	138.64	156.28↑	135.19	123.94	122.43	119.05
	#2	138.64	156.28↑	135.19	126.25	126.76	119.05
$\frac{Max\ Torque}{Isom\ Max\ Torq}$ (%)	#1	35.47	78.14↑	32.61	59.79	30.51	50.51
	#2	35.47	78.14↑	32.61	60.90	31.58	50.51
$\frac{Resisted\ ROM}{ROM}$ (Δ%)	#1	0.79	-8.30	-7.24↓	-4.98↓	1.18	0.00
	#2	0.00	-13.73	-0.45	-7.62↓	24.84	8.70
$\frac{Avg\ Vel\ 50\%}{Avg\ Vel\ 25\%}$ (Δ%)	#1	-33.50		-11.12		-4.65	
	#2	-35.35		-14.89		-17.40	
Max Velocity (deg/sec)	#1	174.4	112.4	182.9	159.1	161.5	159.1
	#2	164.7	108.5	178.1	166.2	182.9	159.1

Secondary Axes

Rot Secondary	#1	--	--	17.2	25.0	56.3	71.9
Max Torq (lb-ft)	#2	--	--	15.6	20.3	71.9↑	75.0
F/E Secondary	#1	110.2	114.9	--	--	110.2↑	112.5
Max Torq (lb-ft)	#2	110.2	114.9	--	--	110.2	110.2
L F Secondary	#1	64.1	64.1	20.3	31.3	--	--
Max Torq (lb-ft)	#2	62.5	67.2	18.8	25.0	--	--

Key

↓ Subnormal, less than -2 Standard Deviations
↑ Supernormal, greater than +2 Standard Deviations
✕ Lateral Flexion Isometric max torque greater than 126 lb-ft

Test Administered By : Jackson T

Signed: _____   Date : _____

B

Figure 9.3 (continued)

upright position. Due to a limitation of the Isostation B-200—the inability to set different resistances during the flexion and extension phase of movement—the lower of the two strength values was used. Subjects were instructed to terminate effort on their own volition. The results showed significant reductions in ROM and velocity in the primary plane and a 100%

OOC Evaluation Results for **Subject B**   *990092320
22-MAR-90

OOC Test	Rotation	Flex/Ext	Lat Flex

Range of Motion

ROM (deg) #1	55.0	86.9	72.6
#2	88.2	90.8	73.5
ROM #2 / ROM #1 (Δ%)	60.36↑	4.49	1.24

Isometric

Max Torque (lb-ft)	50.0	107.8	117.2	117.2

Dynamic

	25%	50%	25%	50%	25%	50%
Avg Torque / Resistance (%) #1	98.33	117.60↑	85.93	99.81	97.93	86.38
#2	99.17	117.60↑	88.52	100.19	95.86	86.38
Max Torque / Resistance (%) #1	130.00	145.60↑	141.11	130.19	172.41↑	142.76↑
#2	130.00	144.00↑	145.56	134.63	177.93↑	142.76↑
Max Torque / Isom Max Torq (%) #1	31.20	72.80↑	32.51	59.98	42.66↑	70.65↑
#2	31.20	72.00↑	33.53	62.03	44.03↑	70.65↑
Resisted ROM / ROM (Δ%) #1	71.14↑	36.91	3.33	-2.22	0.62	-19.88
#2	6.69	-6.69	4.26	1.06	4.91	-29.45↓
Avg Vel 50% / Avg Vel 25% (Δ%) #1	-31.92		-4.82		-22.87	
#2	-38.18		-10.90		-40.10↓	
Max Velocity (deg/sec) #1	137.6	95.0↓	154.4	149.6	149.6	130.6
#2	129.8	95.0	166.2	152.0	185.2	106.9↓

Secondary Axes

Rot Secondary Max Torq (lb-ft) #1	--	--	17.2	23.4	37.5	61.0
#2	--	--	25.0	29.7	40.6	65.6↑
F/E Secondary Max Torq (lb-ft) #1	65.6	53.9	--	--	77.4	84.4
#2	56.3	77.4	--	--	72.7	77.4
L F Secondary Max Torq (lb-ft) #1	71.9	79.7	18.8	23.4	--	--
#2	76.6	81.3↑	23.4	20.3	--	--

Key

↓ Subnormal, less than -2 Standard Deviations
↑ Supernormal, greater than +2 Standard Deviations

Test Administered By : Jackson T

Signed : _____   Date : _____
C

Figure 9.3 (continued)

increase in ROM in the accessory (coronal and transverse) planes. Average endurance time was 40.2 seconds ± 22.3 seconds, with a range of 20 to 118 seconds. The authors suggested that loss of control and coordination that accompanied fatigue may be an important risk factor. The endurance limit is a more useful predictor of incidence and recurrence of low back disorders than the absolute strength values.[70,71]

OOC Evaluation Results for **Subject B**   #990092320
                                                                              22-MAR-90

Demographic Data

Age : 35	Sex : M
Height : 5 ft 10 in	Weight : 145 lbs
Diagnosis : Non-Symptomatic	
Surgical Category : Non-Surgical	
Activity Level Category : Light work	

Resistance Settings

Rotation 25%	:	12 lb-ft
Rotation 50%	:	25 lb-ft
Flex/Ext 25%	:	27 lb-ft
Flex/Ext 50%	:	54 lb-ft
Lat Flex 25%	:	29 lb-ft
Lat Flex 50%	:	58 lb-ft

Abnormal indicators   [0]

	Rotation 25%	Rotation 50%	Flex/Ext 25%	Flex/Ext 50%	Lat Flex 25%	Lat Flex 50%
Average Torque/Resistance		⇑				
Max Torque/Resistance		⇑			⇑	⇑
Max Torque/Isom Max Torque		⇑			⇑	⇑
Isometric Max Torque						
Max Velocity						
Rotation Sec Max Torque						
Flex/Ext Sec Max Torque						
Lat Flex Sec Max Torque						

Non-physiological indicators   [0]

1) not observed
2) not observed
3) not observed
4) not observed
5) not observed
6) not observed
7) not observed

Baseline Rehabilitation Data

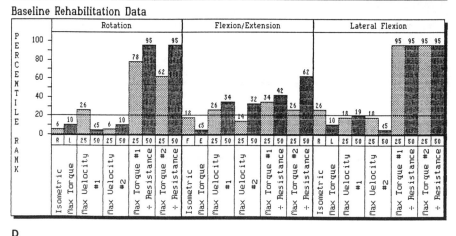

D

Figure 9.3 (continued)

Soft tissues subjected to repetitive loading, due to their viscoelastic properties, demonstrate creep and load relaxation. The loss of precision, speed, and control of the neuromuscular system reduces the soft tissues' ability to protect the weakened passive structures, which may explain many industrial, clinical, and recreational injury mechanisms. The high percentage of Type I back muscle fibers, in addition to better vascularization of these muscle groups, contributes to their superior endurance.[72,73] Physiological studies indicate that at higher muscle utilization ratios (relative loads), fatigue is detected earlier.[74] These results further indicate the necessity of job relatedness of our clinical protocol and show how short duration, maximal isometric testing cannot provide data on these complex functional interactions of strength, endurance, control, and coordination.

One unresolved issue during dynamic testing is how the wealth of information can be presented in a succinct and informative fashion. One approach has been to compare the statistical features of data to the existing normal databases. This is particularly crucial because clinicans do not have the option of comparing results to the "contralateral, asymptomatic joint," as they have with lower or upper extremity joints. Given the large differences between individuals, we recommend comparison be made to job-specific databases. However, given the sparsity of such data, we argue for comparison of functional capacity with job demand.

It should be pointed out that determination of external moments about different joints during a manual material handling task is based on well-established laws of physics. However, the determination of human performance and assessment of functional capacity are based on other disciplines, for example, psychophysics, that are not as exact or well developed as physics. We can describe the job demand easily by analyzing the workers performing the tasks. However, we are unable to predict the ability to perform an arbitrary task based on our incomplete knowledge of functional capacities at the joint levels. In other words, a task is easily decomposed to its demands at the joint level; however, we cannot compose (construct) the arbitrary tasks based on our functional capacity knowledge. For example, holding a load in front of the body with one hand can be resolved into components of flexion and lateral bending for the external moment. However, by combining a given amount of flexion and lateral bending moment we cannot specify the task that produces these components. More critically, knowing the functional capacity of a person in isolated planes, for example, sagittal and coronal planes, does not allow us to extrapolate his ability to perform combined (complex) loading tasks such as simultaneous balancing of a given lateral bending and flexion moment. The challenge of ergonomics and occupational biomechanics is to establish that missing link. Integration of ergonomics and functional analysis depend on the removal of this obstacle.

The enormous degrees of freedom existing in the neuromusculoskeletal system provide the control centers for both kinematic and actuator redundancies. The redundancies provide optimization possibility. Since we can lift an object from point A to point B with infinite postural possibilities, we suggest that certain physical parameters may be optimized for the learned movements. The possible candidates for optimizing objective function are

Table 9.1 Cross-tabulation of different normalized cost functions during 60° of unidirectional trunk flexion and extension with fixed time, $t_f = 1$ second.

	NORMALIZED COST				
	Energy	*Jerk*	*Peak Torque*	*Impulse*	*Work*
FLEXION					
Cost Minimized					
Energy	1.00	2.67	1.34	1.13	1.03
Jerk	1.09	1.00	1.10	1.45	1.05
Peak Torque	1.25	2.08	1.00	1.86	1.18
Impulse	1.01	2.89	1.43	1.00	1.03
Work	1.03	1.84	1.26	1.11	1.00
EXTENSION					
Cost Minimized					
Energy	1.00	12.31	1.46	1.05	1.00
Jerk	1.12	1.00	1.04	1.46	1.05
Peak Torque	1.17	0.29	1.00	1.57	1.18
Impulse	1.04	10.13	1.36	1.00	1.03
Work	1.05	6.28	1.19	1.13	1.00

movement time, energy, smoothness, muscular activities, and so on. This approach, though still in its early stage, may be very important for spine functional assessment. We could compare a given performance to the optimal performance that is predicted by the model (Table 9.1). We have modeled flexion and extension of the trunk and calculated the predicted position and angular velocity of the trunk (Figure 9.4) for different cost functions. Presently, we are validating our model with normal subjects. This approach provides specific goals and gives biofeedback with respect to the individual's performance.

Static versus Dynamic Trunk Strength Measurements

The National Institute for Occupational Safety and Health recommends static, that is, isometric, strength measurement as its current standard for lifting tasks.[75] This was based on evidence that correlated LBP with inadequate isometric strength.[52,76–80] When the measured isometric strength capacity of the individual was less than the strength required by the job, the probability of low back injury was estimated to increase threefold.[52,77]

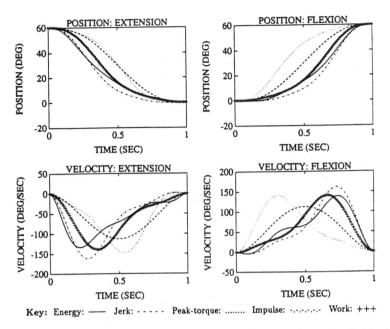

Figure 9.4 Simulation of the optimal trajectories for a unidirectional 60° of trunk flexion and extension using five different cost functions (energy, jerk, peak torque, impulse, and work) with fixed time, $t_f = 1$ second. These profiles can be compared to actual movement profiles and could be used for biofeedback purposes.

Static strength tests have been used as a screening method for selecting workers in strenuous jobs.[77] Himmelstein and Andersson[81] used the industry-based data of Chaffin[52] to predict low back injury in a hypothetical cohort of workers required to do heavy manual material handling. They found that static strength testing has a predictive value ranging from 20% to 53% depending on the incidence rate and test-positivity rate. These poor results do not justify denial of jobs to employees based on static testing.[81]

Battie et al. recently conducted a prospective study to determine the physical risk factors associated with back pain reports among 3,020 aircraft manufacturing employees and found that isometric lifting strength measurements were not predictive of back pain incidence.[82] This was probably because the standard isometric lifting tests used by Battie et al. were not specific for the job. Chaffin et al.[77] and Keyserling[83] have shown that strength tests were more valid if they simulated the demands of the job.

Static strength measurements were also reported to underestimate significantly the loads on the spine during dynamic lifts.[21,84-91] Comparing static and dynamic biomechanical models of the trunk, Leskinen found that, depending on the lifting technique, the predicted spinal loads under static conditions were 33% to 60% less than those under dynamic conditions.[92]

Other studies also showed poor correlations between static lifting performances and maximum acceptable weights of dynamic lifting, as determined by psychophysical tests.[7,93–98] In psychophysical lifting tests, one of the task variables (for example, the weight of the object to be lifted) is under the individual's control. All other variables (for example, the frequency of lift, distance and height of the lift, and size of the object to be lifted) are controlled by the tester. The subject adjusts the amount of weight to be lifted depending on his or her judgment of his or her own strength and endurance level.[99] Troup et al. showed that psychophysical lifting capacity was less in those with previous LBP; however, the measured isometric and psychophysical strengths were a poor predictor of future LBP.[62]

The recruitment patterns of trunk muscles, and thus the internal loading of the spine, is significantly different under isometric and dynamic conditions.[100] Torner et al. found high isometric strength among Swedish fishermen.[101] They found no significant difference in strength between those without pain during the last year and those who had experienced back symptoms during the last seven days. Klein et al. compared spinal mobility and isometric trunk extensor strength with electromyographic spectral analysis for discrimination analysis of low back pain.[102] They found ROM and isometric strength suffered from lower specificity and sensitivity than spectral parameters. Notwithstanding the methodological problems of their study (their discriminant functions were not validated), their concept warrants further investigation.

The widely conflicting results found in the literature regarding the relationship of an individual's strength to the risk of developing LBP may be due to inappropriate modes of strength measurements, that is, lack of job specificity.[69,103] Despite the above controversies, isometric strength testing of the trunk is still widely used, especially in large-scale industrial or epidemiological studies, because it has been standardized and studied prospectively in industry.[81] Compared to trunk dynamic-strength testing protocols, the trunk isometric-strength testing protocols are safer, simpler, and less expensive.[56,104]

In the clinics, isometric strength testing has been used to assess patient progress, treatment efficacy, and the effects of fatigue.[105] If the lumbar muscles can be isolated and tested in different positions through a full range of motion, then multipositional isometric training can be done. This type of training was shown to increase strength throughout the full range of motion in the limb muscles[106–109] and trunk extensor muscles.[37]

Correlations among Different Trunk Strength and Endurance Tests

Parnianpour et al. investigated the correlations between isometric and isokinetic strength and isometric endurance capacity of back muscles in 131 healthy women.[28,110] All subjects underwent a comprehensive test battery that consisted of isometric and isokinetic strength testing of abdominal and back muscles using an isokinetic dynamometer, the Natick upright pull test,[111] and the Sorensen endurance test.[70]

Isometric back and abdominal muscle strength was measured in prone and supine positions. The isokinetic tests were performed in a sitting position at 30 and 60 deg/sec. The Natick upright pull tests were performed in two different postures: (1) upright with the handle at the level of the axilla with a straight back and knees; and (2) upright with the handle 38 cm above the floor with a straight back and bent knees. The Sorensen was performed in the prone position.

A number of correlations exist but are too weak to have significant predictive power. The unexpected results were that isometric endurance had a stronger correlation with isokinetic parameters than with isometric strength parameters. The correlations among isometric tests were low. The isometric results also showed a weak correlation with isokinetic testing modes. There were no significant correlations between maximum isometric flexion and any isometric or isokinetic extension parameter. However, there were strong correlations among the isokinetic extension parameters.

These results are in agreement with those of Thorstensson and Nilsson[36] and Ostering et al.[112] Thorstensson and Nilsson showed that strength measurement is a function of movement velocity, body position, and center of rotation.[36] These data further support the conclusion of Mital and Karwowski, who showed that the use of static strength testing to develop the human performance limit for dynamic tasks is fundamentally incorrect because the inertial forces are ignored.[113] Marras, King, and Joynt[32] and Marras and Mirka[89] showed that muscle recruitment patterns of static and isokinetic movements are drastically different. Another ignored parameter is the time available to complete a lifting task. Hall demonstrated that more rapid lifting significantly increased compressive and shear forces at the L5–S1 level and generated a higher external moment to be balanced by the muscles and other structures of the back.[114]

Strength is a complicated quantity that must be measured through a number of parameters and, based on the 1987 study by Parnianpour et al., static tests cannot be substituted for dynamic tests. McNeill et al.[20] showed isometric trunk muscle strength for back patients and normal individuals to be equal. However, Langrana et al.[31] and Langrana and Lee[115] showed significant differences in isokinetic torque curves between patients and normal individuals, thus demonstrating that dynamic strength and endurance assessments are indispensable.

Correlations among Different Isometric and Dynamic Lifting Tests

Various lifting tests, including static, dynamic, maximal, and submaximal are currently available. Unfortunately, the intercorrelations among these tests are poorly quantified.[60–62,116–118] Parnianpour et al. investigated the intercorrelation among strength measures using various isometric, isokinetic, and isoinertial testing for isolated trunk and multilink coordinated exertions in 43 healthy subjects (21 men and 22 women).[119] The testing equipment used was the Lido Active Back System and the Lido Lift Rehabilitation System. The performance parameters for isokinetic tests were: the peak and average torque, work, joint angle at peak torque for flexion and extension movements at 30 deg/sec, 90 deg/sec, and 120 deg/sec. The parameters of the endurance test at 120 deg/sec were total work performed during one minute of flexion and extension. The peak power, force, and average work were selected for isokinetic lifts during raising and lowering. The selected parameters for isoinertial lifts were the maximum load, peak force, velocity, and acceleration during raising and lowering. They found that the magnitude of correlations varied and no single test emerged as the ideal generic test of choice.

Direct comparison with the existing literature was difficult because no other single study has investigated all the modes of strength testing used in their study. Mayer et al. found very poor correlations among isokinetic lift (at 46 cm/sec and 76 cm/sec) and the isoinertial lifting capacity.[61] The linear correlations ranged from $-.09$ (NS) to 0.62 (p < 0.05). Battie found correlation coefficients to range from 0.5 to 0.85 when comparing isometric strength in arm, leg, and torso lift positions.[103] The correlations were significantly higher among women (from 0.74 to 0.85) than among men (from 0.5 to 0.68).

The results of isometric arm and leg lifts, using the Lido Lift, are higher in the study of Parnianpour et al.[119] compared to the age matched groups in Battie.[103] Zeh et al. also found higher correlation between the arm lift and torso lift for females (r = 0.69) than for males (r = 0.5).[117] They suggested that strength in a different position from the test position was poorly predicted. Due to small sample size, Parnianpour et al. were not able to analyze the effect of gender on the correlations.[119] However, their preliminary results are in agreement with Battie[103] and Zeh et al.[117]

The results of the study by Parnianpour et al. confirm the theoretical prediction that strength will be dependent on the measurement technique.[119] Since muscle action requires external resistance, the effect of muscle action will depend on the nature of the resistance. The implicit assumption is that a generic strength test exists that can be used for preplacing workers (preemployment) and predicting the risk of injury or future occurrence of LBP. The results of their study and others in the literature point to low correlation among various strength measures. In addition, the validity of the injury model for LBP has been questioned and hence, prevention of LBP has proven nearly impossible. The data show prevention of chronicity to be a more effective measure for cost containment. Furthermore, human behavior is highly overdefined and no single parameter should be expected to predict the outcome of a highly complex set of processes in physical and psychosocioeconomic realms.[62,82,120,121]

Hirsch et al. investigated the relationship between performance on lumbar dynamometry and several psychological tests and measures of nonorganic pain behavior in a population with LBP.[122] They concluded that a poor performance on a physical (biomechanical) test may be a form of abnormal illness behavior, which suggests the multifactorial nature of behavior among low back patients. It should be emphasized that the population in the study is relatively chronic with an average of 131.6 days since the injury. Hazard et al. investigated disability exaggeration as a predictor of functional restoration outcomes for chronic LBP patients.[123] They concluded that prescription of intensive multidisciplinary treatment should not be denied based on a patient's individual attributes or the disability exaggeration due to the poor predictive power of treatment outcome.

A recent large prospective industrial study showed that physical measures, including strength, had very low predictive power to explain industrial LBP claims. However, psychosocial factors were determined to be very important in this regard.[103] Before dismissing the need for quantification of trunk function, particularly the strength parameters, critical assessment of the job-relatedness of the strength measures used is needed.[69,77,103] Parnianpour et al. have illustrated how isometric tests can miscalculate the risk assessment of demands on the spine by a given task with respect to a normal population.[69]

Regression analysis was used to model dynamic torque, velocity and power output as a function of resistance level during flexion and extension using the Isostation B-200.[69] Results indicated that dynamic torque was not a good discriminator of the 10th, 50th, and 90th percentile population. (These populations are based on normative data collected by Isotechnologies.) However, velocity and power were shown to effectively discriminate the three populations. Based on these data, it was suggested that during clinical testing, sagittal plane resistance should not be set higher than 60 ft–lbs in order to minimize the internal loading of the spine while taxing trunk functional capacity. The three distributions are completely separable at this resistance level, and higher set resistances will increase the net joint reaction forces on the spine without any added discriminatory advantage. The data in this study were presented in terms of absolute value of resistance rather than normalized with respect to maximum isometric strength as suggested previously.[38]

This presentation of data may be useful for the clinician or ergonomist in evaluating the functional capacity requirements of workplace manual material handling tasks. For example, a manual material handling task that requires 60 ft–lb of trunk extensor strength can be performed by 90% of the population in that database if the required average trunk velocity does not exceed 40 deg/sec, while only 50% could perform the task if the velocity requirement exceeds 70 deg/sec. A few versions of lumbar motion monitors that can record the triaxial motion in the workplace have been used to provide the trunk movement requirements.[125,126]

The more mature debate regarding strength testing should be about which "set" of existing test modes is needed to assess strength capability with respect to job demands. To provide for optimal clinical assessment a "set" of these tests, as dictated by ergonomic analysis of job demands, may be needed. If the task is to flex and extend the trunk at a constant angular velocity with lower extremities stabilized by mechanical means, the selection of the appropriate test should be evident. However, part of the problem is that there is no generic job. The more diverse the demands of a job, the more complex the functional assessment will be. Unless the ergonomists develop tools and techniques that could quantify various dimensions of human performance, existing confusion could prevail and clinicians will have to subject themselves to an asystematic trial-and-error experience with technologies that have evolved on an ad hoc basis. Often these technologies look to their users to provide them a theoretical rationale. The Isokinetics literature is perhaps the best example of this.[127]

The resource-economic paradigm (relating the individual's functional capacities to the task demands) is reflective of the principal goal of ergonomics: fitting the demands of the task to the functional capability of the worker.[128] One of the problems with the present state of the resource-economics paradigm is that fundamental dimensions of performance are assumed to be independent. It is clear during isoinertial lifts that speed, coordination, endurance, and strength are highly correlated. In other words, the assumption that we can tax the system maximally along one dimension of performance to quantify the maximum available resource along that dimension does not hold. During most tests, we perhaps tax more than one dimension and therefore, as more joints are involved and more dynamic tests are utilized, larger contributions of the neuromuscular subsystems will be required. Thus, delineation of the dependent, independent, controlled, and confounding variables becomes more crucial since their numbers rapidly increase with the complexity of the test.

Conclusion

The quantitative methods of trunk performance have been reviewed to unify the existing knowledge of ergonomics and functional assessment. The direction of future research has been identified by pointing to the existing gaps in the literature. Clinical protocols must take into consideration the job demands based on previous ergonomic analysis. Job-related functional evaluation at single or multiple-joint levels have the most promising future. The ergonomists' challenge is to find methods relating jobs to fundamental abilities that can be tested in the clinics. The specificity and sensitivity of the existing biomechanical tests and parameters need more critical attention for both the acute and chronic LBP patient population. It should be realized that objective performance assessment of the trunk contains only partial information about the patient and more prospective randomized clinical and industrial trials are needed to evaluate the relative importance and utility of trunk dynamometers.

References

1. Komi PV: The stretch-shortening cycle and human power output, in Jones NL, McCartney N, and McConas AJ (eds) Human Muscle Power. Champaign, IL: Human Kinetics, 27–39, 1986.
2. Pitman MI, Peterson L: Biomechanics of skeletal muscle, in Nordin M, and Frankel V (eds) Basic Biomechanics of the Musculoskeletal System. Philadelphia: Lea and Febiger, 89–111, 1989.
3. Gowitzke BA, Milner M: Understanding the Scientific Bases of Human Movement, 2nd ed. Baltimore: Williams and Wilkins, 1980.
4. Kroemer KHE, Marras WS, McGlothlin JD, et al: On the measurement of human strength. Int J Industrial Ergonomics 6:199–210, 1990.

*The authors thank Professors Robert Gabriel, Tom Schmitz, Ellen Ross, Margareta Nordin, and Victor H. Frankel for their significant contribution to this chapter. We would like to gratefully acknowledge the financial support of The Ohio State University Research Foundation and the Research Foundation of the Hospital for Joint Diseases Orthopaedic Institute in New York.

5. Hislop HJ, Perrine JJ: Isokinetic concept in exercise. Physical Therapy 47:114–117, 1967.

6. Rodgers MM, Cavanagh PR: Glossary of biomechanical terms, concepts, and units. Phys Ther 64:1886–1902, 1984.

7. Kroemer KHE: An isoinertial technique to assess individual lifting capability. Human Factors, 25:493–506, 1983.

8. Nordin M: Trunk strength and endurance: Measurement techniques, in Weinstein JN and Weisel SW (eds) The Lumbar Spine. Philadelphia: WB Saunders, 859–869, 1990.

9. Smidt G, Herring T, Amundsen L, et al: Assessment of abdominal and back extensor function: A quantitative approach and results for chronic low back patients. Spine 8:211–219, 1983.

10. Plog BA: Fundamentals of Industrial Hygiene, 3rd ed. Chicago: National Safety Council, 862, 1988.

11. Mayhew TP, Rothstein JM: Measurement of muscle performance with instruments, in Rothstein JM (ed) Clinics in Physical Therapy: Measurement in Physical Therapy. New York: Churchill Livingstone, 7:57–102, 1985.

12. Clarke HH: Cable Tension Strength: A Manual, Springfield, MA: Stuart E. Murphy, 1959.

13. Alston W, Carlson KE, Feldman DJ, et al: Quantitative study of muscle factors in the chronic low back syndrome. J Am Geriatric Soc 14:1041–1047, 1966.

14. Nachemson A, Lindh M: Measurement of abdominal and back muscle strength with and without low back pain. Scand J Rehab Med 1:60–65, 1969.

15. Suzuki N, Endo S: A quantitative study of trunk muscle strength and fatigability in low-back pain syndrome. Spine 8:69–74, 1983.

16. Caldwell LS, Chaffin DB, Dukes-Dobos FN, et al: A proposed standard procedure for static muscle strength testing. Am Industrial Hygiene Assoc J 35:201–206, 1974.

17. Chaffin DB: Ergonomics guide for the assessment of human static strength. Am Industrial Hygiene Assoc J 37:505–511, 1975.

18. Troup J, Chapman AE: The flexor and extensor muscles of the trunk. J Biomech 2:49–62, 1969.

19. Addison R, Schultz A: Trunk strength in patients seeking hospitalization for chronic low back disorders. Spine 5:539–544, 1980.

20. McNeill T, Warwick D, Andersson G, Schultz A: Trunk strengths in attempted flexion, extension, and lateral bending in healthy subjects and patients with low-back disorders. Spine, 5:529–538, 1980.

21. Nicolaisen N, Jorgensen K: Trunk strength, back muscle endurance and low back trouble. Scand J Rehab Med 17:121–127, 1985.

22. Jorgensen K: Back muscle strength and body weight as limiting factors for work in the standing slightly-stooped position. Scand J Rehab Med 2:149–153, 1970.

23. Kondraske G, Dervanayagam S, Carmichael T, et al: Myoelectric spectral analysis and strategies for quantifying trunk muscular fatigue. Arch Physical Med Rehab 68:83–110, 1987.

24. Andersson GBJ, Ortengren R, Nachemson A: Quantitative studies of the load on the back in different working postures. Clin Orthop 129:156–164, 1977.

25. Hasue M, Fujiwara M, Kikuchi S: A new method of quantitative measurement of abdominal and back muscle strength. Spine 5:143–148, 1980.

26. Kahanovitz N, Nordin M, Verderame R, et al: Normal trunk muscle strength and endurance in women and the effect of exercises and electrical stimulation. Part 2: Comparative analysis of electrical stimulation and exercises to increase trunk muscle strength and endurance. Spine 12:112–118, 1987.

27. Langrana N, Stover CN: The correlation of clinical and Cybex isokinetic-isometric assessment of back strength and its application to the pre-employment physical examination. Proceedings of the 30th Annual Conference on Engineering in Medicine and Biology 19:187, 1977.

28. Nordin M, Kahanovitz N, Verderame R, et al: Normal trunk muscle strength and endurance in women and the effect of exercises and electrical stimulation. Part 1: Normal endurance and trunk muscle strength in 101 women. Spine 12:105–111, 1987.

29. Smidt G, Amundsen L, Dostal WF: Muscle strength at the trunk. J Orthop Sports Phys Ther 1:165–170, 1980.

30. Davies GL, Gould JA: Trunk testing using a prototype Cybex II isokinetic dynamometer stabilization system. J Orthop Sports Phys Ther 3:163–170, 1982.

31. Langrana N, Lee CK, Alexander H, Mayott CW: Quantitative assessment of back strength using isokinetic testing. Spine 9:287–290, 1984.

32. Marras WS, King AI, Joynt RL: Measurements of loads on the lumbar spine under isometric and isokinetic conditions. Spine 9:176–187, 1984.

33. Mayer TG, Smith S, Keeley J, Mooney V: Quantification of lumbar function. Part 2: Sagittal plane trunk strength in chronic low back patients. Spine 10:765–772, 1985.

34. Mayer TG, Smith S, Keeley J, Mooney V: Quantification of lumbar function. Part 2: Sagittal plane trunk strength in chronic low back patients. Spine 10:765–772, 1985.

35. Thorstensson A, Arvidson, A. Trunk muscle strength and low back pain. Scand J Rehab Med 14:69–75, 1982a.

36. Thorstensson A, Nilsson J: Trunk muscle strength during constant velocity movements. Scand J Rehab Med 14:61–68, 1982b.

37. Graves JE, Pollock ML, Carpenter DM, et al: Quantitative assessment of full range-of-motion isometric lumbar extension strength. Spine 15:289–294, 1990.

38. Parnianpour M, Nordin M, Kahanovitz N, Frankel V: The triaxial coupling of torque generation of trunk muscles during isometric exertions and the effect of fatiguing isoinertial movements on the motor output and movement patterns. Spine 13:982–992, 1988.

39. Parnianpour M: Modeling of trunk muscles recruitment during isometric exertions. IEEE Eng Med Biol 10:2, 51–54, 1991.

40. Dumas GA, Poulin MJ, Roy B, et al: A three-dimensional digitization method to measure trunk muscle lines of action. Spine 13:532–541, 1988.

41. MacIntosh JE, Bogduk N: The detailed biomechanics of the lumbar multifidus. Clin Biomech 1:205–231, 1986.

42. MacIntosh JE, Bogduk N: The morphology of the lumbar erector spinae. Spine 12:656–668, 1987a.

43. Rab G, Chao E, Stauffer R: Muscle forces analysis of the lumbar spine. Orthop Clin North Am 8:193–199, 1977.

44. Yettram AL, Jackman MJ: Structural analysis for the forces in the human spinal column and its musculature. J Biomed Eng 4:118–124, 1982.

45. Dumas GA, Poulin MJ, Roy B, et al: Orientation and moment arms of some trunk muscles. Spine 16:293–303, 1991.

46. Buchalter D, Parnianpour M, Viola K, et al: Three-dimensional spinal motion measurements. Part 1: A technique for examining posture and functional spinal motion. J Spinal Disord 1:279–283, 1989.

47. Pearcy M, Portek I, Shepherd J: Three-dimensional x-ray analysis of normal movement in the lumbar spine. Spine 9:294–297, 1984.

48. Pearcy M, Portek I, Shepherd J: The effect of low-back pain on lumbar spinal movements measured by three-dimensional x-ray analysis. Spine 9:150–153, 1985.

49. Panjabi M, Yamamoto I, Oxland T, Crisco J: How does posture affect coupling in the lumbar spine? Spine 14:1002–1011, 1989.

50. Tan JC: The effect of sagittal-standing trunk posture on temporal and amplitude recruitment patterns, and triaxial torques of trunk muscles during isometric trunk extension. (Doctoral dissertation, New York University). Ann Arbor, MI: University Microfilms International, 1991.

51. Parnianpour M, Campello M, Sheikhzadeh A: The effect of posture on triaxial trunk strength in different directions: Its biomechanical consideration with respect to incidence of low-back problem in construction industry. Int J Industrial Ergonomics 8:3, 279–288, 1991.

52. Chaffin DB: Human strength capability and low back pain. J Occup Med 16:248–254, 1974.
53. Westgaard RH: Measurement and evaluation of postural load in occupational work situations. Eur J Appl Physiol 57:291–304, 1988.
54. Kroemer KHE, Marras WS: Evaluation of maximal and submaximal static muscle exertions. Human Factors, 23:643–653, 1981.
55. Yang JF, Winter DA: Electromyography reliability in maximal and submaximal isometric contractions. Arch Physical Med Rehab 64:417–420, 1983.
56. Kroemer KHE: Ergonomics, in Plog BA (ed) Fundamentals of Industrial Hygiene, 3rd ed. Chicago: National Safety Council, 283–334, 1988.
57. Chaffin DB, Baker WH: A biomechanical model for analysis of symmetric sagittal plane lifting. AIIE Transactions 2:16–27, 1970.
58. Schultz A, Andersson G: Analysis of loads on the lumbar spine. Spine 6:76–82, 1981.
59. Asmussen E, Poulsen E, Rasmussen B: Quantitative evaluation of activity of the back muscle in lifting. Communications from Danish National Association of Infantile Paralysis 21:3–14, 1965.
60. Mayer T, Barnes D, Kishino N, et al: Progressive isoinertial lifting evaluation: I. A standardized protocol and normative database. Spine 13:993–997, 1988a.
61. Mayer T, Barnes D, Nichols G, et al: Progressive isoinertial lifting evaluation: II. A comparison with isokinetic lifting in a disabled chronic low-back pain industrial population. Spine 13:998–1002, 1988b.
62. Troup J, Foreman T, Baxter C, Brown D: The perception of back pain and the role of psychophysical tests of lifting capacity. (1987 Volvo Award in Clinical Sciences). Spine 7:645–657, 1987.
63. Bryant JT, Stevenson JM, French SL, et al: Four factor model to describe an isoinertial lift. Ergonomics 33:173–186, 1990.
64. Ross EC: The effect of resistance level on muscle coordination patterns and truncal velocity, acceleration and deceleration during isoinertial trunk extension. Unpublished Doctoral Thesis, New York University, 1991.
65. Schmitz TJ: The effect of direction and resistance level on muscle coordination patterns and truncal velocity, acceleration and deceleration during unidirectional isoinertial trunk flexion and extension of healthy males. Unpublished Doctoral Thesis, New York University, 1992.
66. Gabriel RJ: The effect of direction and resistance level on muscle coordination, movement patterns and motor output during repetitive isoinertial trunk flexion and extension of healthy males. Unpublished Doctoral Thesis, New York University, 1992.

67. Ross EC, Parnianpour M, Martin D: Timing and amplitude of trunk activity during extension under varying loading conditions. Spine, In press, 1993.

68. Deutsch S. OOC Back Evaluation System. Isotechnologies, Inc. Hillsborough, NC, 1991.

69. Parnianpour M, Tan J, Hofer HO, Sheikhzadeh A: Toward a multivariate normal distribution analysis in evaluation of trunk performance during nonregulated (isoinertial) movement. International Society for Study of Lumbar Spine, Boston, June 13–17, 61, 1990.

70. Biering-Sorensen F: Physical measurements as risk indicators for low back trouble over a one-year period. (1983 Volvo Award in Clinical Science.) Spine 9:106–119, 1984.

71. Jorgensen K, Nicolaisen T: Trunk extensor endurance: Determination and relation to low back trouble. Ergonomics 30:259–267, 1987.

72. Bende-Peterson F, Mork AL, Nielsen F: Local muscle blood flow and sustained contraction of the human arm and back muscles. Eur Appl Physiol 34, 1975.

73. Zhu XA, Parnianpour M, Nordin M, Kahanovitz N: Histochemistry and morphology of erector spinae muscles in lumbar disc herniation. Spine 14:391–397, 1989.

74. Parnianpour M, Nordin M, Moritz U, Kahanovitz N: Correlation between different tests of trunk strength, in Buckle P (ed) Musculoskeletal Disorders at Work. New York: Taylor & Francis, 1987.

75. National Institute for Occupational Safety and Health (NIOSH): Work Practices Guide for Manual Lifting (DHHS Publication No. 81–122). Washington, DC: U.S. Government Printing Office, 1981.

76. Andersson GBJ: Epidemiologic aspects on low back pain in industry. Spine 6:53–60, 1981.

77. Chaffin DB, Herrin GC, Keyserling WM: Preemployment strength testing: An updated position. J Occup Med 20:403–408, 1978.

78. Chaffin DB, Park K: A longitudinal study of low back pain as associated with occupational weight lifting factors. Am Industrial Hygiene Assoc J 34:513–525, 1973.

79. Keyserling WM, Herrin GD, Chaffin DB: Isometric testing as a means of controlling medical incidents on strenuous jobs. J Occup Med 22:332–336, 1980.

80. Schultz A, Haderspeck K, Warwick D, Portillo D: Use of lumbar trunk muscles in isometric performance of mechanically complex standing tasks. J Orthopedic Res 1:77–91, 1983.

81. Himmelstein JS, Andersson GBJ: Low back pain: Risk evaluation and preplacement screening, in Himmelstein JS, Pransky GS (eds) Occupational Medicine: State of the Art Review: Worker Fitness and Risk Evaluations 3:255–269, 1988.

82. Battie M, Bigos SJ, Fisher LD, et al: Isometric lifting strength as a predictor of industrial back pain reports. Spine 14:851–855, 1989.
83. Keyserling WM: Isometric strength testing in selecting workers for strenuous jobs (Doctoral dissertation, The University of Michigan). Ann Arbor, MI: University Microfilms International, 1979.
84. Buseck M, Schipplein OD, Andersson GBJ, Andriacchi TP: Influence of dynamic factors and external loads on the moment at the lumbar spine in lifting. Spine, 13:918–921, 1988.
85. Foreman T, Baxter C, Troup J: Ratings of acceptable load and maximal isometric lifting strength: The effects of repetition. Ergonomics 27:1283–1288, 1984.
86. Freivalds A, Chaffin DB, Garg A, Lee KS: A dynamic biomechanical evaluation of lifting maximum acceptable loads. J Biomechanics 17:251–262, 1984.
87. Marras WS: Predictions of forces acting upon the lumbar spine under isometric and isokinetic conditions: A model-experiment comparison. Int J Industrial Ergonomics 3:19–27, 1988.
88. Marras WS, Mirka GA: Muscle activities during asymmetric trunk angular accelerations. J Orthopaedic Res 8:824–832, 1990.
89. Marras WS, Mirka GA: A comprehensive evaluation of trunk response to asymmetric trunk motion. Spine 17:318–326, 1992.
90. Smith J, Smith L, McLaughlin T: A biomechanical analysis of industrial manual material handlers. Ergonomics, 25:299–308, 1982.
91. Wood GA, Hayes KC: A kinetic model of intervertebral stress during lifting. Br J Sports Med 8:74–79, 1974.
92. Leskinen TPJ: Comparison of static and dynamic biomechanical models. Ergonomics 28:289–291, 1985.
93. Garg A, Mital A, Asfour S: A comparison of isometric strength and dynamic lifting capability. Ergonomics 23:13–27, 1980.
94. Garg A, Sharma D, Chaffin D, Schmidler J: Biomechanical stresses as related to motion trajectory of lifting. Human Factors 25:527–539, 1983.
95. Kamon E, Kiser D, Pytel J: Dynamic and static lifting capacity and muscular strength of steelmill workers. Am Industrial Hygiene Assoc J 43:853–857, 1982.
96. Khalil T, Asfour S, Waly S, Genaisy A: A comparative study of static and dynamic lifting tasks. Proceedings of the 28th Annual Meeting of the Human Factors Society, 595–599, 1984.
97. Mital A, Karwowski W, Mazouz A, Orsarh E: Prediction of maximum acceptable weight of lift in the horizontal and vertical planes using simulated job dynamic strengths. Am Industrial Hygiene Assoc J 47:288–292, 1986.

98. Poulsen E: Prediction of maximum loads in lifting from measurement of back muscle strength. Progressive Therapy 1:146–149, 1970.

99. Snook SW: Psychophysical acceptability as a constraint in manual working capacity. Ergonomics 28:327–330, 1985.

100. Marras WS, Reilly CH: Networks of internal trunk-loading activities under controlled trunk motion conditions. Spine 13:661–667, 1988.

101. Torner M, Zetterberg C, Hansson T, Lindell V: Musculoskeletal symptoms and signs and isometric strength among fishermen. Ergonomics 33:1155–1170, 1990.

102. Klein AB, Snyder-Mackler L, Roy SH, DeLuca CJ: Comparison of spinal mobility and isometric trunk extensor forces with electromyographic spectral analysis in identifying low back pain. Phys Ther 71:445–454, 1991.

103. Battie M: The reliability of physical factors as predictors of occurrence of back pain reports. A prospective study within industry. Doctoral Dissertation, Gottenburg University, 1989.

104. Stevenson JM, Bryant JT, French SL, et al: Dynamic analysis of isoinertial lifting technique. Ergonomics 33:161–172, 1990.

105. Roy SH, Deluca CJ, Casavant DA: Lumbar muscle fatigue and chronic lower back pain. Spin 14:992–1001, 1989.

106. Graves JE, Pollock ML, Jones A, et al: Specificity on limited range of motion variable resistance training. Med Sci Sports Exercise 21:84–89, 1989.

107. Kahanovitz N, Nordin M, Verderame R, et al: Normal trunk muscle strength and endurance in women and the effect of exercises and electrical stimulation. Part 2. Comparative analysis of electrical stimulation and exercise to increase trunk muscles strength and endurance. Spine 12:112–118, 1987.

108. Kamon E, Kiser D, Pytel JL: Dynamic and static lifting capacity and muscular strength of workers. Am Ind Hyg Assoc J 43:853–857, 1982.

109. Kulig K, Andrews JG, Hays JG: Human strength curves. Exercise Sport Sci Rev 12:417–466, 1984.

110. Parnianpour M, Shecter S, Moritz U, Kahanovitz N: Back muscle endurance in response to external load. Proceedings of American Society of Biomechanics. University of California Davis, 167–168, 1987.

111. Knapik JJ, Vogel JA, Wright JE: Measurement of isometric strength in an upright pull at 38 cm. Natick, MA, U.S.A. Medical Research Institute of Environmental Medicine, Report number T3/81, April 1, 1981.

112. Ostering R, Bates B, James S: Isokinetic and isometric torque relationship. Arch Phys Med Rehabil 58:254–259, 1977.

113. Mital A, Karwowski W: Use of simulated job dynamic strength (SJDS) in screening workers for manual lifting task. Proceedings of Human Factors Society, 29th Annual Meeting, 513, 1985.

114. Hall, S: Effect of attempted lifting speed on forces and torque exerted on the lumbar spine. Med Sci Sports Exerc 15:440–444, 1985.
115. Langrana N, Lee, CK: Isokinetic evaluation of trunk muscles. Spine 9:171–175, 1984b.
116. Freivalds A, Fotouki DM: Comparison of dynamic strength as measured by the Cybex and Mini-Gym isokinetic dynamometers. Int J Industrial Ergonomics 1:189–208, 1987.
117. Zeh J, Hansson T, Bigos SJ, et al: Isometric strength testing: Recommendations based on a statistical analysis of the procedure. Spine 11:43–46, 1986.
118. Beimborn DS, Morrissey MC: A review of literature related to trunk muscle performance. Spine 13:665–660, 1988.
119. Parnianpour M, Hasselquist L, Aaron A, Fagan L: The intercorrelation among isometric, isokinetic, and isoinertial muscle performance during multi-joint coordinated exertions and isolated single joint trunk exertion. Sixth Annual Meeting of the North American Spine Society (NASS), Keystone, CO, July 31-August 3, 1991.
120. Hadler NM: Clinical Concepts in Regional Musculoskeletal Illness. Orlando: Grune & Stratton, 1987.
121. Hadler NM: Disabling backache in France, Switzerland, and Netherlands: Contrasting sociopolitical constraints on the clinical judgment. J Occup Med 31:823–831, 1989.
122. Hirsch G, Beach G, Cooke C, et al: Relationship between performance on lumbar dynamometry and Waddel Score in a population with low-back pain. Spine 16:1039–1043, 1991.
123. Hazard RG, Bendix A, Fenwick JW: Disability exaggeration as a predictor of functional restoration outcomes for patients with chronic low-back pain. Spine 16:1062–1067, 1991.
124. Snijders CJ, Van Riel MD, Nordin, M: Continuous measurements of spine movements in normal working situations over periods of 8 hours or more. Ergonomics 30:639–653, 1987.
125. Marras WS, Sandhaker LR, Lavender SA: Three-dimensional measures of trunk motion components during manual material handling in industry. Proceedings of Human Factors Society 33rd Annual Meeting, Santa Monica, CA, 662–666, 1989.
126. Ostering R: Isokinetic dynamometry: Implication for muscle testing and rehabilitation. Ex Sport Sci Rev 14:45–80, 1986.
127. Kondraske GV: Quantitative measurement and assessment of performance, in Smith RV, Leslie JH (eds) Rehabilitation Engineering. Boca Raton: CRC, 101–125, 1990.

10 □□□ □□□ □□□

Case Reports: Use of Trunk Dynamometers in the Management of Patients with Spinal Disorders

This chapter reports, in a case study format, a variety of clinical experiences in which the technology of isokinetic trunk dynamometers has been used as part of a successful treatment regimen in the management of patients with spinal disorders. Although the clinical situations were limited to the technology of two specific manufacturers—Cybex Division of Lumex, Inc., Ronkonkoma, NY and Isotechnologies Inc., Hillsborough, NC—the rehabilitation experiences demonstrated the potential effectiveness of this mode of evaluation and therapeutic exercise, which should be equally applicable to other types of spinal dynamometers. It is also important to note that the patient experiences reflected an integrated approach to the management of spinal disorders; the patients received treatment that was appropriate to their individual case and not just trunk exercise. The following case reports may be valuable for spinal clinicians who wish to add trunk dynamometry to their existing repertoire of patient care services.

Kent E. Timm

CASE REPORT 1: QUADRUPLE SPINAL SURGERY PATIENT*

History

A 45-year-old 175 lb male was referred February 20, 1987, for rehabilitation following four separate lumbar surgeries: a right L5 laminec-

---

*By Kent E. Timm.

tomy in January 1982, a right L3 laminectomy in January 1983, a left L-4 laminectomy in August 1984, and a failed L4–L5 interbody fusion in July 1986. The patient complained of a continuous dull ache throughout his lumbar spinal region with intermittent pain peripheralization into both lower extremities. The pain did not adhere to a specific pattern of response to positions, postures, and activities and prohibited the patient from sitting and from riding in a car for prolonged periods of time. Previous attempts at symptom remediation included moist heat, ultrasound, massage, diathermy, traction, TENS, electrical stimulation, joint mobilization, myofascial release, Williams exercise, back school program, McKenzie technique, biofeedback, epidural injection, and acupuncture treatments, none of which resulted in a lasting relief of the patient's symptoms. The patient was on a restricted duty occupational status at his workplace, an automobile foundry, and was complying with a physician prescribed regimen of multiple pain medications.

Evaluation

The patient presented with a right lower extremity antalgic gait and demonstrated a general diminishment of lumbar mobility in all motion planes secondary to pain. Specific mobility testing revealed an empty, painful end-feel at all lumbar segmental levels. Manual muscle testing revealed fair grade strength in all muscle groups of the paravertebral, abdominal, hip, and leg regions, accompanied by a pain magnification response on resistive testing. Straight leg raising yielded a positive test response at 40 degrees in both lower extremities. The Waddell battery of clinical tests[1] revealed a score of 1 on the 5-point scale, indicating the absence of inappropriate illness behavior at the time of the initial evaluation. The patient consented to an isokinetic test on the Cybex Trunk Extension Flexion (TEF) dynamometer and produced muscle torque values of 49 foot-pounds and 31 ft-lbs for spinal flexion and 38 ft-lbs and 18 ft-lbs for spinal extension at the test speeds of 30 and 60 degrees per second (deg/sec), respectively, through a 40 degree range of motion. The specific arc of patient movement was from a position of 90° vertical to the position of 40° forward from vertical (0° to 40°). The test procedure paralleled a standard isokinetic spinal assessment method (Table 10.1), but testing was ceased above the speed of 60 deg/sec for the patient could not generate any form of muscle torque output. The evaluation process yielded a physical therapy diagnosis for the patient of a spinal deconditioning syndrome secondary to multiple surgeries.

Table 10.1   Isokinetic Test Formats[6]

Spinal Dynamometry in the Sagittal (Flexion/Extension) and Transverse (Left/Right Rotation) Planes				
Warm-Up:	10 minutes of aerobic activity at 300–600 kgm/min			
	3 submaximal plus 1 maximal trial at each speed			
Testing:	Speed*	30	60	90	120	150
	Reps	04	04	04	04	20
	Rest	20–60 seconds between speeds			
	ROM	patient determined; available			
	Intensity	patient determined; comfortable			

*isokinetic speeds in deg/sec

Treatment

Formal rehabilitation began on February 21, 1987. The patient was placed on a program of isokinetic exercise, cardiovascular conditioning, and cold modalities on a three treatment sessions per week basis, complemented by a home exercise program. The isokinetic program consisted of a velocity spectrum format which involved 10 repetitions of a spinal flexion/extension cycle at the speeds of 30, 60, 90, 120, and 150 deg/sec through the patient's 0 to 40 degree range of tolerable spinal motion. The patient was asked to perform the motions of flexion and extension at each step of the speed progression-regression sequence at his self-determined level of comfort, with emphasis on the extension component, and was allowed up to 1 minute of rest between exercise speeds. The spinal arc of motion was progressed by up to 5° per session, depending on the patient's levels of comfort and tolerance, toward the functional goal of movement from 15° extension to 90° flexion. The isokinetic program is summarized in Table 10.2.

Isokinetic exercise was integrated with a clinical regimen of cardiovascular conditioning, cryotherapy, and a home exercise program. Cardiovascular training preceded the isokinetic exercise routine and consisted of a 20-minute period of aerobic-type exercise on a bicycle ergometer or walking, depending on the patient's comfort level, within the work intensity range of 300 to 600 kilogram-meters per minute. Aerobic walking was also incorporated into the patient's home exercise program, which was performed on a daily basis. Cryotherapy followed cardiovascular and isokinetic exercise and involved a 20-minute period of lumbar cooling, with topical ice packs, while the patient was positioned in a prone-on-elbows posture supported by pillows. As a complement to the clinical treatments and in addition to the aerobic walking program, the patient's home exercise routine consisted of procedures designed to enhance lumbar muscle strength, spinal movement

Table 10.2 Velocity Spectrum Exercise[6]

Stage	Speed*	Repetitions	Rest Period
1	30	10	20–60 sec
2	60	10	20–60 sec
3	90	10	20–60 sec
4	120	10	20–60 sec
5	150	20	20–60 sec
6	120	10	20–60 sec
7	90	10	20–60 sec
8	60	10	20–60 sec
9	30	10	20–60 sec
	Intensity: patient determined; comfortable		
	ROM: patient determined; available		

*isokinetic speeds in deg/sec

capacities, and vertebral segmental control. The individualized program incorporated the exercise treatment philosophies of the McKenzie and muscle stabilization training methods.[2,3,4] The patient was also supplied with a lumbar roll for use as a spinal support during sitting and driving activities.

Progress

On March 5, 1987, the patient produced 75, 49, 20, and 4 ft-lbs of spinal flexion torque and 62, 44, 15, and 2 ft-lbs of spinal extension torque at the respective speeds of 30, 60, 90, and 120 deg/sec on reevaluation with the isokinetic dynamometer. Such improvements occurred even though the patient's subjective pain complaint was largely unchanged. Treatment was progressed by increasing the intensity of the patient's exercise effort at each stage of the isokinetic velocity spectrum sequence, but never to the point of exceeding the patient's relative level of comfort or tolerance. The rehabilitation program of isokinetic exercise, cardiovascular training, cryotherapy, and home procedures was retained for the duration of the patient's clinical treatment experience.

On March 19, 1987, the patient reported a decrease in his symptoms which accompanied the ability to take short automobile trips without experiencing back pain. He produced flexion torque values of 111, 82, 56, 39, and 11 ft-lbs and extension torque values of 108, 81, 63, 38, and 9 ft-lbs at the respective isokinetic test speeds of 30, 60, 90, 120, and 150 deg/sec on reassessment of his functional status through spinal dynamometry. On March 26, 1987, the patient reported that he had diminished the dosage of his pain medication by one-half and that he was now able to sleep for continuous nightly periods of six to eight hours without relying on sleeping pills. The patient demonstrated flexor torques of 141, 125, 92, 80, and 55 ft-lbs and extensor torques of 155, 135, 106, 87, and 62 ft-lbs at the standard isokinetic test speeds.

On April 2, 1987, the patient reported that he was completely without back pain for the first time in four years and that his occupational activity level had been ungraded to light duty from a restricted status. At isokinetic testing, the patient produced outputs of 170, 152, 137, 100, and 73 ft-lbs for spinal flexion and spinal extensor torques of 187, 161, 143, 112, and 81 ft-lbs across the standard speed spectrum. At this point the patient began a gradual reduction of the clinical program, consisting of two weeks of twice weekly treatments followed by two weeks of one treatment session per week, while the home exercise program remained intact.

On May 1, 1987, the patient produced spinal flexor muscle torques of 248, 228, 196, 177, and 142 ft-lbs and spinal extensor muscle torques of 292, 258, 211, 184, and 155 ft-lbs at the standard testing speeds. The patient reported that he was totally free of spinal symptoms and that he had been able to successfully resume all of his normally required occupational activities, as well as his usual activities of daily living, without any restrictions. At this point the patient was formally discharged from rehabilitation with the advice to maintain the performance of the home exercise program on a daily basis, to report his progress on a biweekly basis, and to report for follow-up isokinetic tests on a monthly basis. An orthopedic reevaluation before discharge revealed normal values for lumbar motion[5] and normal dermatomal and myotomal functions.

Follow-up isokinetic tests were performed on the patient in June, July, and August 1987 as an ongoing assurance that his rehabilitation program had been successful. On all occasions the patient produced muscle torque values for both flexion and extension that were within 5 ft-lbs of his performance on May 1, 1987. In addition, he had remained gainfully employed and completely asymptomatic since the end of the clinical program. Overall, treatment consisted of 19 sessions over a period of 42 calendar days, followed by the phase-out period of 6 treatment sessions over 26 calendar days, for a program total of 25 sessions over 68 calendar days from the point of initial evaluation through the date of discharge.

References

1. Waddell G, McCulloch JA, Kummel E, et al: Nonorganic physical signs in low-back pain. Spine 5:117–125, 1980.
2. DiMaggio A, Mooney V: The McKenzie program: Effective exercise against back pain. J Musculoskel Med 4:63–74, 1987.

3. McKenzie RA: The lumbar spine: Mechanical diagnosis and therapy. Waikanae, New Zealand: Spinal Publications, 1981.
4. White AH, Anderson R: Conservative Care of Low Back Pain. Baltimore, Williams and Wilkins, 1991.
5. Timm KE: Back injuries and rehabilitation. Baltimore, Williams and Wilkins, 1990.

CASE REPORT 2:
SPINAL STENOSIS PATIENT*

History

A 50-year-old 160 lb male patient was referred for spinal rehabilitation on February 26, 1990, following spinal surgery on February 5, 1990, for the decompression of lumbar spinal stenosis. The stenotic condition affected the L4 and L5 segmental vertebral levels and was believed to be congenital. Before spinal surgery, the patient had experienced a gradual progression of lower back pain over a 30-year period, which started as a vague and intermittent discomfort about age 20 but finalized as a constant and sharp pain sensation. The patient's symptoms did not directly affect his occupational performance as an accountant but did curtail recreational athletic pursuits as a distance runner and cross-country skier. Following the successful surgery, which had been classified as routine and uneventful by the patient's neurosurgeon, the patient was placed on a regimen of pain medication and gentle flexibility exercises, as per the direction of his referring physician, before the start of clinical rehabilitation activities.

Evaluation

The patient presented with primary complaints of lower back stiffness accompanied by a general sensation of lumbar muscle weakness. The patient did not report any real experience of lower back pain since the time of surgery. Neurological testing revealed normal dermatomal, deep tendon reflex, and proprioceptive responses in the patient's lumbar region and in both lower extremities. Manual muscle testing showed good to normal grades of strength in the T12–S2 myotomal distributions of the spine and both legs. Functional motion testing revealed normal movement capabilities for spinal extension, left and right rotation, and left and right lateral flexion accompanied by a flexion limitation at 70° forward bending. Isokinetic test-

---

*By Kent E. Timm.

Table 10.3 Isokinetic Data Reduction[6]

Motion	Flexion/Extension/Rotation				
Speed	30	60	90	120	150
Parameter	PT%BW	PT%BW	AP%BW	AP%BW	AP%BW
Parameter	TW%BW	TW%BW	TW%BW	TW%BW	TW%BW
Parameter					ER

Parameter Key: PT%BW = peak torque percent body weight; AP%BW = average power percent body weight; TW%BW = total work percent body weight; ER = endurance ratio.

INTERPRETATION

Average Performance Ratio (APR) = Mean of Parameters
APR = (PT%BW + PT%BW + AP%BW + AP%BW + AP%BW + TW%BW
  + TW%BW + TW%BW + TW%BW + TW%BW) / 11
Average Performance Deficit (APD) = 100% − APR

EXAMPLE

Motion	Flexion				
Speed	30	60	90	120	150
Data	100	95	72	100	105
Data	75	72	67	55	50
Data					64

APR = (100 + 95 + 72 + 100 + 105 + 75 + 72 + 67 + 55 + 50 + 64) / 11
  = 78%
APD = 100% − 78%
  = 22%

ing, using the Cybex TEF spinal dynamometer and a standardized assessment method (Table 10.1), demonstrated a 70% deficit of spinal extensor muscle performance capacity. The data reduction paralleled the process format that appears in Table 10.3. The evaluation process yielded a physical therapy diagnosis of functional instability of the lumbar spine, secondary to spinal extensor muscle insufficiency.

Treatment

Rehabilitation began on the same date as the initial evaluation, February 26, 1990, and consisted of cardiovascular conditioning and isokinetic exercise procedures complemented by a home treatment program. Cardiovascular conditioning consisted of bicycle ergometry at the work intensity level of 600 kilogram-meters per minute for 20 minutes' duration. An additional aerobic stimulus through fitness walking was integrated into the patient's home program. Isokinetic exercise, which duplicated the general format displayed in Table 10.2, consisted of a velocity spectrum approach across the speed spectrum of 30 to 150 deg/sec. Exercise intensity was determined by the patient's perceived levels of comfort and tolerance to the isokinetic activity. Activity was accomplished through an initial range of motion of 0° to 70° flexion, but progressed toward the goal of increasing the arc of motion by 5° for both spinal flexion and extension with each treatment session. The clinical program was undertaken on a three sessions per week basis and was complemented by a home program of fitness walking and muscle stabilization exercises that was performed by the patient on a daily basis.[1]

Progress

The patient's treatment program continued, progressing within his self-determined levels of comfort and tolerance, until a reevaluation session on March 7, 1990. At that time, the patient continued to demonstrate normalcy of dermatomal and myotomal functions, but also showed a spinal flexion mobility capability of 80°. In addition, the patient demonstrated a normal spinal extensor muscle performance capacity, and a 0% functional deficit on isokinetic testing. The patient also denied the experience of any form of lower back pain and also stated that he had been able to resume all desired recreational athletic activities without disability. The patient was discharged from rehabilitation, since he had attained a functional level of spinal flexion mobility along with a normal degree of muscle performance ability, but was monitored through biweekly reports and monthly follow-up isokinetic tests. Isokinetic tests performed in April, May, and June 1990 demonstrated normal levels of spinal muscle performance capabilities. The patient's entire clinical program comprised a total of 5 treatment sessions over 11 calendar days.

References

1. White AH, Anderson R: Conservative Care of Low Back Pain. Baltimore, Williams and Wilkins, 1991.

CASE REPORT 3: MICRODISCECTOMY PATIENT*

History

A 38-year-old female was referred from rehabilitation on January 2, 1990, following a microdiscectomy surgical procedure on December 12, 1989, for remediation of an L5 herniated nucleus pulposus. The patient's dis-

---

*By Kent E. Timm.

cal disorder was of rapid insidious onset in November 1989, but was not able to be directly linked to any form of predisposing injury, traumatic episode, or occupational activity. Since the time of surgery, the patient had been without general complaints, denied any experience of spinal pain or discomfort, and had successfully returned to her normal occupational duties as a seamstress. The patient did, however, have a feeling of relative muscle weakness throughout her lower lumbar spine, which prompted the referral for spinal rehabilitation from her neurosurgeon.

Evaluation

The patient was subjected to a standard orthopedic physical therapy evaluation consisting of mobility, neurological, and manual muscle testing procedures. On functional mobility testing the patient demonstrated normal movement capabilities for the motions of spinal extension, left and right lateral flexion, and left and right rotation, but did demonstrate a limitation of spinal flexion, the specific arc being from anatomical neutral to 65° forward bending. Neurological testing procedures revealed normal dermatomal, deep tendon reflex, and proprioceptive responses throughout the lumbar spinal region and the bilateral lower extremities. Straight leg raising was negative for discal and for dural irritation. Manual muscle testing revealed good grade muscle strength throughout the T12–S2 segmental myotomal distributions.

The patient also consented to spinal muscle performance testing on the Cybex TEF and Trunk Rotation (TORSO) isokinetic dynamometers under the standardized assessment protocols (Table 10.1). Isokinetic testing, using the data reduction scheme shown in Table 10.3, demonstrated performance deficits of 52% for the spinal extensor muscles, 40% for the spinal flexor musculature, and 10% for the left spinal rotator muscle group. The evaluation process yielded a physical therapy diagnosis of functional instability of the lumbar spine, secondary to general muscle insufficiency.

Treatment

Starting on the same day as the initial evaluation, January 2, 1990, the patient began a therapeutic program of cardiovascular conditioning activity, progressive resistance training, and isokinetic exercise undertaken on a two sessions per week clinical basis. Cardiovascular conditioning consisted of aerobic exercise on a bicycle ergometer for 20 minutes' duration at a work intensity load of 600 kilogram-meters per minute. Aerobic activity was followed by progressive resistance exercise on weight training machines for

Table 10.4 DAPRE Format[5,6]

Set	Load	Repetitions
1	0.50 (x)	10
2	0.75 (x)	6
3	(x)	maximum
4	adjusted	maximum

Repetitions: Set 3	*Load: Set 4*	*(x): Next Session*
0–2	decrease 2–5 kg	decrease (x) 2–5 kg
3–4	decrease 0–2 kg	(x) unchanged
5–7	(x) unchanged	increase (x) 2–5 kg
8–12	increase 2–5 kg	increase (x) 5–7 kg
13 +	increase 5–7 kg	increase (x) 7–9 kg

the spinal flexor, spinal extensor, and spinal rotator muscle groups. The weight lifting program followed the DAPRE format[1,2] detailed in Table 10.4.

Isokinetic exercise followed the velocity spectrum rehabilitation format, which has been described in the previous case reports and appears in Table 10.2. The patient exercised in progressive and regressive cycles across a speed spectrum of 30 to 150 deg/sec at a self-determined, comfortable intensity through a self-determined, comfortable arc of spinal motion. Exercise involved both the Cybex TEF and TORSO dynamometers for sagittal and transverse plane activity, respectively. The clinical program was complemented by a home program of aerobic walking and muscle stabilization exercises similar in nature to those in the previous case reports.[3]

Progress

Treatment progressed at the patient's level of tolerance until a reevaluation session on January 15, 1990, when the isokinetic dynamometry procedures were repeated. Testing revealed that the patient's functional movement capacity had improved to 70° flexion from the initial evaluation finding of 65°. In addition, the patient's spinal flexor muscle performance deficit had diminished to 16% from 40% while the spinal extensor muscle performance deficit had dropped from 52% to 26%. Isokinetic testing also demonstrated that spinal rotatory muscle functions had normalized; the 10% deficit in left rotation had been reduced to 0%.

The clinical program continued biweekly until another reevaluation session on January 30, 1990. At that time the patient demonstrated normalcy of spinal movement capabilities in each of the sagittal, frontal, and transverse motion planes as well as the complete absence of muscle performance deficits for the spinal flexor, extensor, and rotator muscle groups on isokinetic testing. In addition, the patient denied any form of pain or spinal discomfort and reported the continued ability to engage in occupational and recreational activities without limitations. The patient was formally discharged from treatment, but was instructed to report her status on a biweekly basis and to report back to the clinic for follow-up spinal tests on a monthly basis to assure the success of her rehabilitation. All postdischarge reports were noneventful and all follow-up isokinetic tests continued to demonstrate the absence of a performance deficit in the patient's spinal muscle groups. The entire rehabilitation program consisted of 9 clinical sessions over a period of 29 calendar days.

References

1. Timm KE: Back injuries and rehabilitation. Baltimore, Williams and Wilkins, 1990.
2. Knight KL: Knee rehabilitation by the daily adjustable progressive resistance exercise techniques. Am J Sports Med 7:336–337, 1979.
3. White AH, Anderson R: Conservative Care of Low Back Pain. Baltimore, Williams and Wilkins, 1991.

CASE REPORT 4: OBJECTIVE MONITORING OF EXERCISE RESULTS*

History

The patient was a 34-year-old 5 ft 9 in. 219 lb male referred for evaluation and treatment of chronic low back pain. The patient's initial evaluation was performed in February 1986, approximately 22 months after his original injury. The patient worked as a truck driver for a waste disposal company. He reported injuring himself opening the back of the truck and pushing on the door. At the time of the injury, he had felt a "pop" in his lower back and was unable to continue working. He was initially seen by an orthopedic surgeon who recommended physical therapy. The patient-reported treatment by the physical therapist consisted of heat, ultrasound, and massage. Within approximately 4 months, the patient reported returning to work with some continuing discomfort. He reported reinjuring himself 7 or 8 months later when sawing wood at work. Since that time, the patient had been treated only with medication and rest and had not returned to work. X-rays and a

---

*By Brian P. D'Orazio.

myelogram were negative. The patient changed physicians and was then sent by his new attending physician to our office.

Physical Examination

The patient initially presented, on standing examination, in a 10° forward incline position with a protuberant abdomen and an erythematous area in the right low back area. The patient indicated this was the area of his chief complaint and the erythema had been present for at least the past year. He was unaware of any reason for the erythema. The patient was tender to palpation directly over this area which extended between about T12 and L3 and covered an area about 4 inches by 4 inches. Even light touch to this area provoked symptoms. The patient's movements were severely limited with no more than 10° of movement in any direction. On seated examination, he was unable to forward bend more than 5°, and while lying supine he was unable to tolerate hip flexion, either actively or passively, past 60°. Straight leg raising was limited to 10° bilaterally, with normal reflexes and no alterations in dermatomal sensation or myotomal strength. The cause for the erythema was never determined during the patient's treatment, but eventually resolved. My assessment was that the patient was severely deconditioned, and that the area of his chief complaint had reacted much like a reflex sympathetic dystrophy.

Treatment and Subsequent Examinations

The patient was started on a range of motion program which, at the first session, increased his active hip flexion to 110° and increased his forward bending to approximately his ankles while seated. The patient was also able to assume an erect posture following a backward bending program. The area of erythema was treated with brief intense TENS, cryotherapy, and gradual desensitization to touch. At his third appointment, a baseline test was performed on the Isostation B100. Against the maximum resistance offered by the B100, the patient was able to produce peak torques of 45 lb-ft for flexion, 51 lb-ft for extension, 20 lb-ft for rotation to the right, 16 lb-ft for rotation to the left, 57 lb-ft of right lateral flexion, and 26 lb-ft of left lateral flexion (Figures 10.1A,B,C). As are demonstrated in the first portion of his test, force productions are well below anticipated norms. At this time, normal values based on in-office testing of males indicated that peak values for flexion and extension should be approximately 145 lb-ft with approximately 70 lb-ft of rotation and 75 lb-ft of lateral flexion. Significant limitations in the Isostation B10 limited accurate isometric testing.

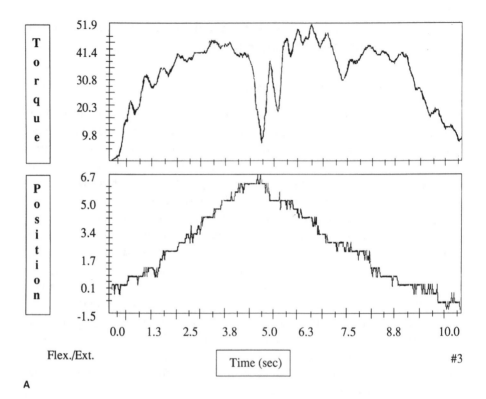

Flex./Ext.

Time (sec)

#3

A

Figure 10.1A Isostation B100 tests for flexion and extension. Resistance is set at 100 lb-ft. The patient forward bends approximately 6° during this test which is the result of a gradual hydraulic release even though the set resistance is above the patient's force production. The second movement is extension. The graph demonstrates the patient's difficulty in attaining and maintaining a peak torque. Peak torque values are therefore approximate.

Figures 10.1D and 10.1E represent the patient's movement test for sagittal and horizontal plane movements, respectively. The patient's resistance during this phase of testing was such that it permitted him to move freely. The patient's range at this stage in his clinical treatment was still limited as is demonstrated by his positional data. An analysis of the patient's torque curves demonstrates erratic force production choices for both sagittal and horizontal plane movement.

The patient was not seen again for one month because of insurance problems. When treatment resumed, the patient's movements were less coordinated and he had resumed some of his forward bent posturing. Movements were more limited than before the patient's one-month absence. The patient's treatment and reconditioning program was resumed and he was retested on the Isostation B100 about 2 weeks later. The patient's torque pro-

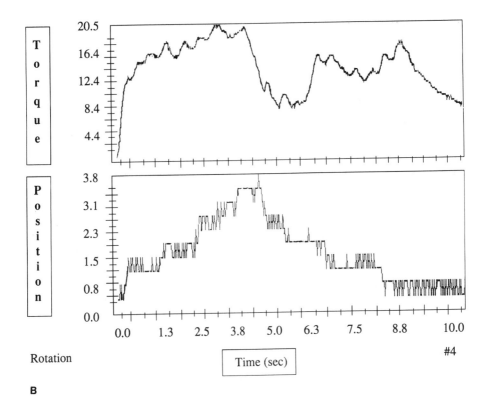

Rotation

Time (sec)

#4

B

Figure 10.1B Rotation against maximum resistance of 63 lb-ft. Again there is some baseline movement; however, the patient's movement velocity is below 1 deg/sec. Again, the patient demonstrates an inability to achieve and maintain a peak torque. Values are approximately 20 lb-ft for right rotation and approximately 16 lb-ft for left rotation.

duction remained essentially unchanged for flexion and extension but increased to about 63 lb-ft for lateral flexion to each side, and increased to about 60 lb-ft of left rotation with 37 lb-ft of right rotation. I continued progressing the patient in his reconditioning program and retested him within 4 weeks. By the patient's next test, his torque values for flexion had increased to 109 lb-ft, with 126 lb-ft of extension, and about 66 lb-ft of lateral flexion torque. Rotational torque was more variable with 46 lb-ft in right rotation and 40 lb-ft in left rotation. His values in general were considered to be about 20% to 30% below normal with the exception of lateral flexion, which was considered to be essentially within normal limits. The patient was progressed to a walking program, and much of his exercise program was performed at home. In the office, he was exercised on the Isostation B100 and on the Fitron, along with treatments including progressive mobilization of the lum-

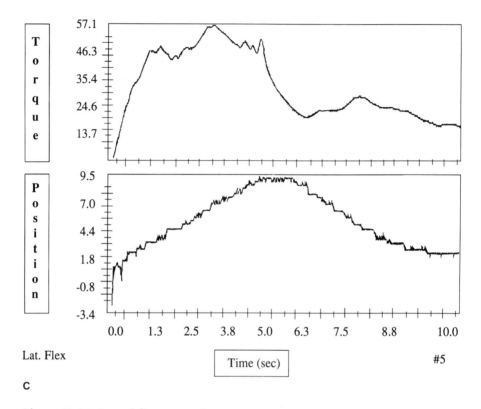

Lat. Flex   Time (sec)   #5

C

Figure 10.1C Lateral flexion on the Isostation B100 is tested at a resistance of 63 lb-ft. Peak torque values were about 57 for right lateral bending and about 26 lb-ft for left lateral bending.

bar spine and lower extremities. The patient was again tested on the B100 about 4 weeks later with marginal gains in performance. It was determined that the patient could then return to light duty, which was specifically defined for the patient and his employer. The patient reported an exacerbation of symptoms 2 weeks after returning to work. This exacerbation seemed to set the patient back for about 3 to 4 weeks. During this time, he was continuing to work on an exercise program at home and was involved in a reconditioning program at the office, but his office program did not replicate his home program. During the next 2 months, he had several exacerbations of symptoms which he could not relate to any specific event. Because of the exacerbations and forgetting to reschedule this individual for a retest, it was about 2 months before his follow-up test on the B100. Testing at follow-up indicated a slight decrease in the patient's force production and movement capabilities.

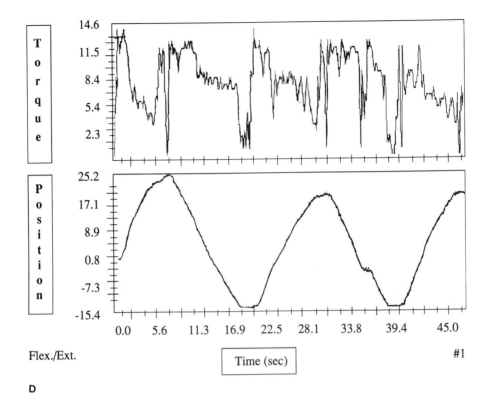

Figure 10.1D Flexion and extension movement tests on the Isostation B100. The first movement is flexion (indicated by a positive positional deflection), followed by extension (indicated by a negative positional deflection).

Conclusions

During the two months that the patient was not retested on the B100, he indicated that he was faithfully pursuing his home therapeutic exercise program. After his last test, I determined that perhaps this was not the case and began more closely monitoring his exercises by having him pursue his entire home exercise program in the office, in addition to his reconditioning program. After testing the patient again in 4 weeks, his values had increased substantially and, in most areas, were within normal limits. The patient was then released to full-duty work and was followed up 4 weeks later with a repeat test on the Isostation B100 that indicated peak torques of 133 lb-ft for flexion, 145 lb-ft for extension, approximately 70 lb-ft for rotation, and approximately 76 lb-ft for lateral bending in each direction (Figures 10.2A,B,C). These were determined to be essentially normal values and in-

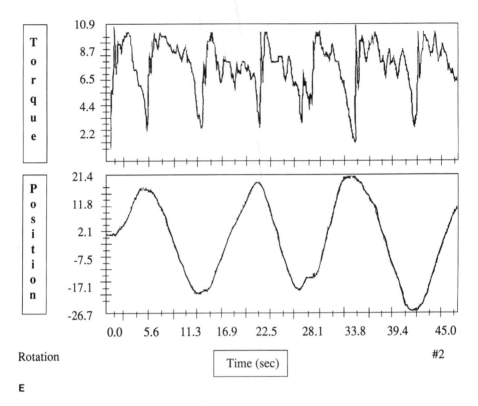

E

Figure 10.1E Rotational movement on the Isostation B100. Rotation to the right is represented as a positive positional deflection and rotation to the left is represented as a negative positional deflection on the patient's graph.

dicated a substantial gain in a fairly short period of time. Movement testing is represented in Figures 10.2D and 10.2E. These tests were performed at 80 lb-ft resistance for flexion and extension and 30 lb-ft for rotation. The patient's movement velocity had clearly increased as had the patient's total movement excursion for both sagittal and horizontal plane movements. It was apparent that the patient was benefiting from a more supervised program, which he later admitted forced him to be consistent with his exercises. The patient was successful in returning to full-time employment at his previous job, and at 1 year he had continued to be successful in that job.

By failing to continuously monitor the patient on the B100, I was unable to monitor objective progress, but rather, relied on the patient's subjective information. This proved to be inaccurate and prolonged the patient's course of rehabilitation. The correction in his performance pattern was readily evident once he was followed up with consistent testing on the B100, expediting the patient's return to full-duty employment. Since this incident, I have monitored patients more consistently in their programs by retesting at about 4-

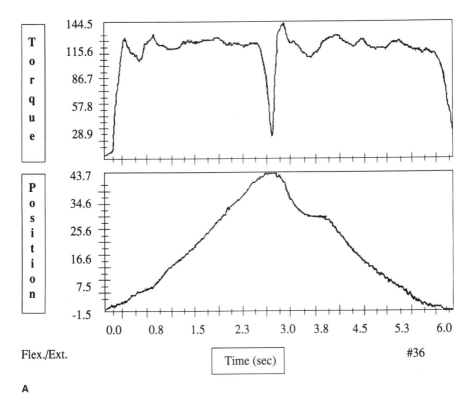

A

Figure 10.2A Flexion and extension tested at a maximum resistance of 100 lb-ft on the Isostation B100. Note the difference in shape of the patient's curves. At this time the patient is able to achieve and maintain his peak torque.

week intervals and find that programs progress at a faster pace with consistent monitoring. This especially seems to be true for chronic pain patients with negative neurological testing who have been out of work for long periods of time and present primarily with severe deconditioning.

CASE REPORT 5: ROLE OF THE ISOSTATION B-200 IN ASSESSING MAXIMUM VOLUNTARY EFFORT*

History

In April 1992, a 42-year-old male was re-referred to my office with complaints of chronic low back pain and lower extremity pain. The patient originally injured his back in July 1986 while working as a firefighter, dragging a bag of refuse up a hill. I first treated the patient from December

---

*By Barbara Danahy Ehman.

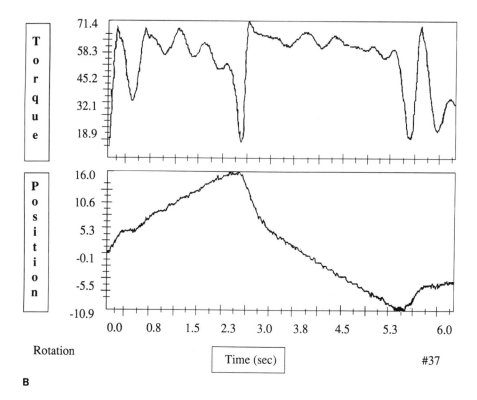

Figure 10.2B Rotational testing at a maximum resistance setting of 63 lb-ft for the Isostation B100. The first torque production is representative of right rotation and the second of left rotation. Note that the patient's torque production is somewhat smoother to the left but in both cases, there is a substantial change in the patient's force production and in the quality of that force production by comparison to his initial test.

1988 until April 1989. Before December 1988, he had been treated in two other physical therapy clinics. Prior testing prescribed by the attending orthopedist and neurosurgeon included several CAT scans, three myelograms, two EMGs, and an MRI scan. All tests failed to show any surgically treatable problem. My original treatment program in 1988 consisted of soft tissue and joint mobilization, ultrasound, ice, and a progressive resistive exercise program. After 4 months of treatment, the patient was able to perform 3 sets of 10 to 15 repetitions of each exercise at the following levels: 60 lb. bench press, 40 lb. lateral trunk bend, 60 lb. leg extension, 60 lb. leg curl, 75 lb. seated row, 75 lb. pull down, and 25 lb. dead lift. I was unable to progress the patient's dead lift beyond 25 lbs., even though this appeared to be submaximal, because of consistent complaints of pain with this activity. There were also inconsistencies noted between his performance levels with exercise and his

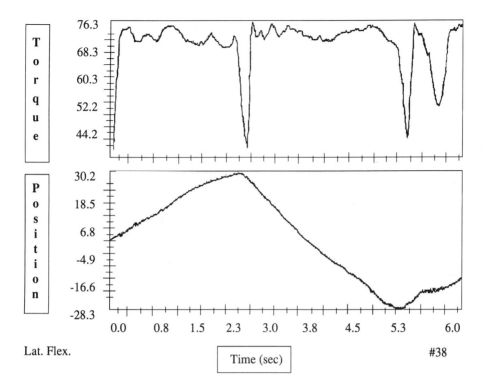

Figure 10.2C Lateral flexion at a maximum setting of 63 lb-ft for the Isostation B100. Torque production again is much higher than previously and is sustained at near peak torque values throughout the tests.

observed functional capabilities. At discharge, I recommended that the patient work with a 25 lb. lifting restriction from floor to waist height. All other constraints fell within the guidelines listed based on his exercise capabilities. He expressed an interest in woodworking which was also documented.

In the fall of 1989, the patient was referred to a pain management clinic, not having returned to work. He subsequently underwent a series of nerve blocks which reportedly provided him minimal symptomatic relief. He continued with medication and pain management counseling for the next year. The patient was then referred to another clinic for work hardening. He participated in this program for six weeks, but reported no symptomatic relief or functional change at its conclusion.

In August 1991, the patient lifted a basket of clothes while at home and felt a sudden "pop" in his back with pain in his left leg, opposite his original injury. He was referred to another neurosurgeon. New tests indicated a bulged

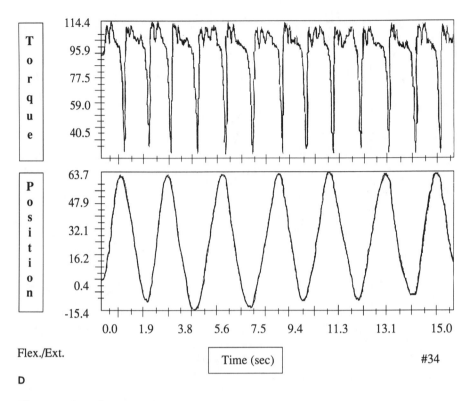

Flex./Ext.

Time (sec)

#34

D

Figure 10.2D Flexion and extension movement at 80 lb-ft resistance for the Isostation B100. The patient's movement velocity, total range of motion, and peak torques have all increased substantially.

lumbar disc. A discectomy was performed in February 1992. He was subsequently re-referred to my office for work hardening and reconditioning.

Evaluation

Subjectively, the patient's chief complaint was pain radiating from the lower back into the right posterior thigh. He reported some symptoms of "tingling" bilaterally in the lower back and right hip with numbness below the knees bilaterally. His symptoms were aggravated with prolonged sitting, standing, or walking. He indicated that there had been a significant reduction in left lower extremity symptoms following surgery, but no change in right lower extremity symptoms which had been present since 1986.

Objectively, the patient presented with no significant postural deviations. Active range of motion in the trunk was moderately limited in all planes. Lower extremity flexibility was within normal limits. Manual muscle testing of all lower extremity myotomes was within normal limits. Pal-

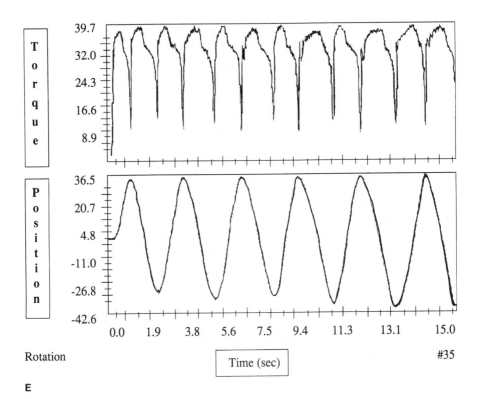

Rotation   Time (sec)   #35

E

Figure 10.2E Rotational movement testing at 30 lb-ft on the Isostation B100. Both right and left rotation demonstrate substantial increases in total excursion as well as in movement velocity and peak torque production.

pation produced tenderness over the surgical site and bilaterally in the longissimus thoracis and iliocostalis lumborum.

Of the four Waddell tests conducted for evaluation of nonorganic physical signs, three were positive. The standing axial loading test and the standing rotation test both elicited complaints of low back pain. A seated dural test was negative at 90° bilaterally in contradiction with a supine straight leg raise test which was positive on the left side at 50° and on the right side at 40°.

Assessment/Plan

My assessment revealed subjective complaints of weakness and paresthesia but no objective evidence of neurological deficits. There were minor areas of diffuse soft tissue tenderness and some limitation of active range of motion. An assumption of deconditioning was made based on evaluation of the patient's tolerance to exercise and prolonged presurgical and postsurgical inactivity. A postsurgical MRI indicated no evidence of disc herniation. The physician's letter to the patient stated, "The bottom line of all of this is that there is no major problem in your back and you can proceed with full activities according to the schedule that we have already worked out." I therefore made a recommendation that the patient be placed in the work reconditioning program and be assigned to the pain management director for further evaluation and goal setting.

The purpose of the work reconditioning and pain management program is to minimize disability associated with chronic pain through the identification of nonorganic barriers to recovery. The work reconditioning and pain management program is typically 4 to 6 weeks long and emphasizes the patient's responsibility in restoring function while deemphasizing symptomatic treatment. The program combines progressive resistive exercise, aerobic conditioning, and behavioral modification. There is a strong emphasis on patient education. Written materials, audiotapes, and videos are frequently selected as an adjunct to care. The pain management director and physical therapist work together to assist the patient in goal setting and determine the plan of action to achieve the set goals.

The pain management director assists in identifying barriers to recovery through a multifactorial collection of data from psychometric testing, a structured personal interview, performance testing, and behavioral observation. In screening for gross psychopathology, the Beck's Depression Inventory revealed scores that indicated mild mood disturbances. The patient's scores on the McGill's Pain Questionnaire indicated that he would be unlikely to respond to physical therapy. His self-report of pain intensity on the three 10 cm Continuous Pain Scales indicated a nonphysiological response (see Chapter 6, Managing Symptom Magnification). In response to the inquiry about the patient's goals, he reported that his goals were, "to play golf, go fishing, receive retirement disability, and not work." Documented observations indicated uncooperative behavior in many aspects of the program.

Dynametric Testing

The Jamar Hand Dynamometer was used to record maximum isometric strength. The results indicate that while males age 40 to 44 typically record values between 113 and 117 lbs. of force at handle position #2, the patient scored between 55 and 63 lbs. of force. The plotted data formed a normal bell shape curve. Isokinetic lower extremity testing also indicated highly variable results with repeat testing. A difference of 40 lb-ft between Test #1 and Test #2, performed on the same day, was documented with testing of the right quadriceps musculature. Trunk testing was performed on the Isostation B200. The isoinertial tests on the B200 are by far the most sophisticated and in many ways the most interesting evaluation of maximum voluntary effort.

Table 10.5   Movement Tests

		Primary Axis		Secondary Axis		Secondary Axis	
		Flexion	Extension	Lateral Flexion		Rotation	
				Right	Left	Right	Left
A	Torque	29.3	24.5	4	—	6	—
	Velocity	**85.5 max**	44.9 avg.	—	—	—	—

		Rotation		Flexion	Extension	Lateral Flexion	
		Right	Left			Right	Left
B	Torque	13.3	15.6	**12–20**	—	**34.4**	**37.5**
	Velocity	81.4 max.	35.6 avg.	—	—	—	—

		Lateral Flexion		Rotation		Flexion	Extension
		Right	Left	Right	Left		
C	Torque	21.0	18.8	5–10	—	—	3
	Velocity	78.4 max.	35.1 avg.	—	—	—	—

Torque measurements in lb-ft.

Velocity in °/sec.

Set resistance for Flexion/Extension—25 lb/ft.

Set resistance for Rotation—15 lb-ft.

Set resistance for Lateral flexion—20 lb-ft.

The Isostation B200 is a tri-axial machine that measures range of motion, velocity of movement and torque production. Because of the unique tri-axial system, data is collected from the primary axis as well as secondary axes. In this case study, the patient presented with highly variable results in all phases of his testing. Two separate test sessions were conducted during the same day. The first series of tests included dynamic as well as isometric tests, and the second set of tests included repeat isometric tests for flexion/extension and rotation as well as an endurance test for flexion/extension.

During the flexion/extension movement test, the patient produced a maximum velocity in flexion of 85.5 deg/sec at 25 lb-ft resistance (Table 10.5). The movement test took approximately 15 seconds to perform. During the endurance test, which lasted 120 seconds, the patient kept a constant velocity of 97.4 deg/sec at a set resistance of 38 lb-ft. The patient's peak torque and peak velocity productions were fairly stable with a slight increase in velocity noted over the 120-second test. The patient also never entered into any substitution pattern in the secondary axes even on an intermittent basis. The data indicated no significant fatigue by the end of the 120-second test. When comparing the endurance test results to the initial flexion/extension movement test, the patient's results clearly demonstrated sub-maximal efforts.

In comparing Test #1 and Test #2 for isometric flexion and extension, the patient produced a maximum torque of 37.5 lb-ft for flexion with a 27.3

Table 10.6   Isometric Tests

		Primary Axis		Secondary Axis		Secondary Axis	
		Flexion	*Extension*	*Rotation*		*Lateral Flexion*	
				Right	Left	Right	Left
A	Test #1	**37.5 max** 27.3 avg.	79.7	2	—	5	—
	Test #2	**75.0 max** 38.3 avg.	89.1	1	—	4	—

		Rotation		*Lateral Flexion*		*Flexion*	*Extension*
		Right	Left	Right	Left		
B	Test #1	23.4	31.3	5–10	5–15	—	**28.1 max.** 12.7 avg.
	Test #2	31.3	34.4	8–17	14–21	—	**28.1 max.** 11.5 avg.

		Lateral Flexion		*Rotation*		*Flexion*	*Extension*
		Right	Left	Right	Left		
C	Test #1	**56.3**	**43.8**	4	10	—	6–10 avg.
	Test #2	Not Performed					

Torque measurements in lb-ft.

lb-ft average for Test #1 compared to a 75 lb-ft maximum effort for flexion with a 38.3 lb-ft average torque production in Test #2 (Table 10.6). In addition to the inconsistencies between Test #1 and #2 for isometric flexion, the patient's maximum torque output during the endurance test was consistently 42.7 lb-ft. The patient's force production of 37.5 lb-ft for isometric flexion in Test #1 was clearly submaximal. Torque production for isometric extension was more stable at 79.7 lb-ft in Test #1 compared to 89.1 lb-ft in Test #2 (Table 10.6,A).

When evaluating and comparing movement patterns in the primary and secondary axes, typical couplings are expected based on normal biomechanics. During flexion/extension, little coupling is expected in the secondary axes. Rotation and lateral flexion, however, are typically associated with well-defined coupled motions in the secondary axes. In testing the patient's rotational movement, lateral flexion torque was 34.4 lb-ft to the right and 37.5 lb-ft to the left. There was also a consistent coupling into flexion of 12 to 20 lb-ft (Table 10.5,B). This combination of flexion with rotation is the typical coupling pattern expected during rotation (Figures 10.3A,B,C,). During the isometric rotation test, the patient used an atypical pattern of movement, coupling rotation with extension (Figures 10.4A,B,C). The patient produced a consistent extension force of 28.1 lb-ft for both Test #1 and Test #2 (Table

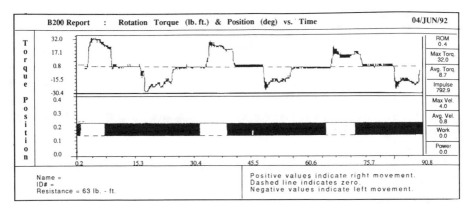

Figure 10.3A Isometric rotation torque in the primary axis; expected coupling pattern.

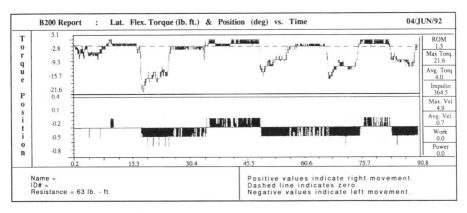

Figure 10.3B Lateral flexion torque in the secondary axis of the rotation isometric test; expected coupling pattern.

10.6,B). From a kinesiological standpoint, it would be difficult to imagine a movement strategy that would use the back extensors to contribute to rotation.

In comparing lateral flexion in the primary and secondary axes, the patient was able to produce 37.5 lb-ft for lateral flexion in the secondary axis while performing the rotation movement test (Table 10.6,B), whereas his maximum isometric torque in the primary axis for lateral flexion was only 43.8 lb-ft to the left and 56.3 lb-ft to the right (Table 10.6,C). The lateral flexion isometric tests would seem to be submaximal. It was also noted that the patient demonstrated no significant coupling pattern into rotation or flexion/extension during the lateral flexion isometric or movement tests. Considering all factors, the patient's test results indicated a submaximal effort and

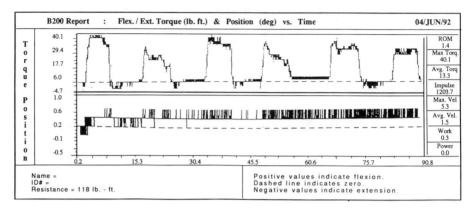

Figure 10.3C Flexion/extension torque in the secondary axis of the rotation isometric test; expected coupling pattern.

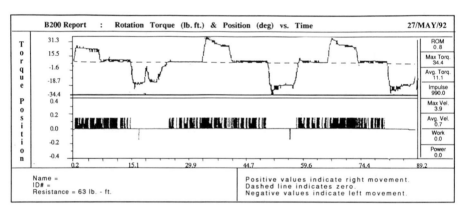

Figure 10.4A Isometric rotation torque in the primary axis; atypical coupling pattern.

therefore could not be considered a valid indicator of the patient's maximal capabilities during testing on the Isostation B200.

Recommendations

The results of multiple dynametric tests, psychometric tests, and a functional capacity evaluation were used to make recommendations for the patient's future employment status. The patient's functional capabilities were clearly documented along with specific guidelines for lifting restrictions and tolerance to standing, walking, and sitting activities. No further physical therapy treatments were recommended based on a perceived level of maximum benefit of treatment and the patient's long history of extensive medical intervention and present attitudes toward recovery.

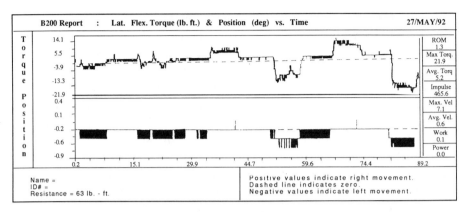

Figure 10.4B Lateral flexion torque in the secondary axis of the rotation iso-metric test; atypical coupling pattern.

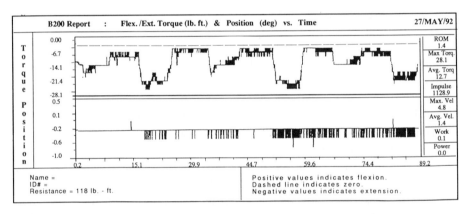

Figure 10.4C Flexion/extension torque in the secondary axis of the rotation isometric test; atypical coupling pattern.

CASE REPORT 6: VALIDATION OF TREATMENT USING THE ISOSTATION B100*

History

A 44-year-old male was referred for evaluation and treatment of chronic low back pain on June 20, 1985. The original injury occurred when lifting weights while in high school. A second injury occurred when being tackled during a collegiate football drill. At that time, a myelogram was performed and the patient was diagnosed with a herniated L4–L5 disc. The

---

*By Paul L. Lysher.

patient elected to terminate football activities and declined surgical intervention. While working at a summer job, between the patient's junior and senior years in college, a low back strain was sustained as a result of lifting. Symptoms were alleviated with medication. Since that time, there had been intermittent low back pain. In 1983, the patient again sought medical attention from a local orthopedic surgeon during an acute exacerbation. Lumbar X-rays were taken and the patient again was diagnosed with a herniated disc. The patient reported increased symptoms primarily after yard work or while lifting when either hunting or fishing. A primary factor in seeking medical attention again in 1985 was apprehension over a possible progressive and debilitating spinal problem. The patient had several weeks of increased symptoms before he was referred for physical therapy evaluation and treatment. His general health was excellent with no other pertinent medical history.

Evaluation

At the time of the initial examination, the patient's chief complaint was low back pain with either prolonged sitting or forward bending. Pain was reported to be greatest in the morning and decreased as the day progressed.

There was a positive distraction test of the left sacroiliac joint. A long sitting test was positive, with the left lower extremity being long in supine and increasing in length when the patient assumed a long sitting position. While standing, the patient was able to forward bend extending his fingertips to the inferior patellar region before experiencing pain. Extension and lateral flexion were within normal limits and pain-free. Pain and increased tone were palpated throughout the left pelvic girdle musculature, most notably the iliopsoas and hip external rotators. In addition, there was tenderness over the left sacroiliac joint and left pubic tubercle.

Neurological testing revealed equal and symmetrical lower extremity reflexes. All lower extremity myotomes were within normal limits. There appeared to be no dermatomal lower extremity sensory deficits. The patient reported decreased discrimination to light touch throughout the lateral aspect of the left lower extremity.

Following the initial examination, the patient's back function was tested on the Isostation B100 (see Figures 10.5 through 10.8). Velocity testing was performed against a moderate resistance and the patient was requested to move through full pain-free ranges of motion. Maximum resistance testing was utilized within the capability of the testing apparatus, that is, no lock-outs were available.

In summary, the patient presented with a left posteriorly rotated ilium and painful trunk flexion. Soft tissue involvement was localized to the left iliopsoas and hip external rotators. There were no positive neurological findings.

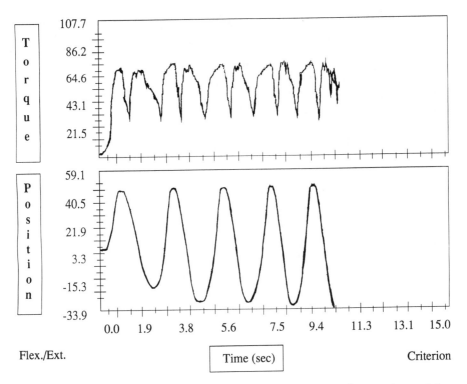

Figure 10.5 Maximum torque values produced for flexion and extension; original test June 20, 1985.

Treatment and Subsequent Reexaminations

After testing on the Isostation B100, a manipulation was performed for the left sacroiliac joint. Following treatment, pelvic mechanics were normalized and the patient was able to forward bend extending his fingertips to the ankle region without a report of pain. A long sitting test was negative. Ultrasound was administered to the left SI joint and external rotators. Instruction was given in a home flexibility program with emphasis on the iliopsoas, quadratus lumborum, hip abductors/external rotators, and hamstrings.

Four days after the initial examination, the patient was reevaluated. At that time, there was no complaint of pain except for "tightness" in the low back region. Pelvic mechanics and trunk range of motion remained normal. A long sitting test was negative. There was minimal tenderness over the left hip external rotators. Instruction was given in a progressive flexibility program and an aerobic exercise program was initiated consisting of both bicycling and walking.

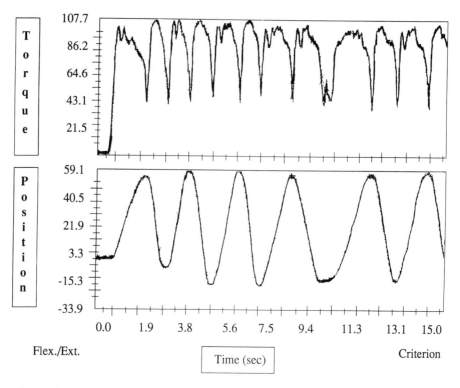

Figure 10.6 Maximum torque values produced for flexion and extension; follow-up test on July 17, 1985.

On July 2, 1985, the patient had no complaints of either back or hip pain. There was a continued report of low back "stiffness." Pelvic mechanics and trunk range of motion remained normal. A long sitting test was negative. Soft tissue palpation was now also negative. The patient was instructed in a trunk reconditioning exercise program primarily to improve back extensor function.

On July 17, 1985, the patient returned for a follow-up examination and retesting on the Isostation B100. Most dramatically, maximum torque values for flexion and extension were increased from 70 to 107 lb-ft (see Figures 10.5 and 10.6, respectively). Rotational values were increased from 34 to 44 lbs-ft (Figure 10.7). Test results for lateral flexion were unchanged (Figure 10.8). After only several weeks, these objective changes documented by the Isostation B100 gave clear evidence as to the efficacy of the treatment. The patient's final examination was performed on July 22, 1985. He had no complaints of either hip or low back pain. Trunk range of motion was within normal limits. Pelvic mechanics were normal. Soft tissue palpation was negative. Accessory motion testing of the lumbar spine failed to reveal any significant joint dys-

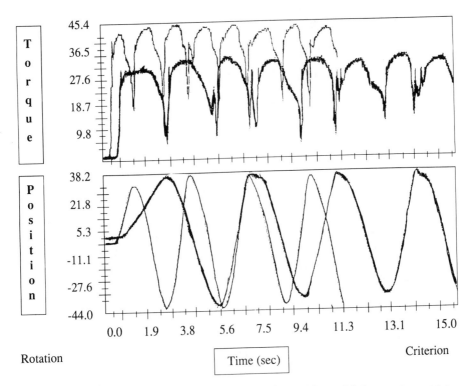

Figure 10.7 Maximum torque values produced for right and left rotation; original test June 20, 1985 and follow-up test on July 17, 1985.

function. Instruction was given in a progressive trunk reconditioning exercise program with further emphasis on extension. The patient was discharged on a home program.

Conclusions

Over the past 7 years, the patient reports that back symptoms are controlled with modification of activity and/or with stretching exercises. Symptoms are primarily experienced with prolonged sitting or after golfing. The patient reports that he is confident he can control his symptoms and feels further treatment is unnecessary at this time.

In summary, the Isostation B100 was an invaluable tool to objectify back function and to correlate changes in signs and symptoms with an increase in movement velocity and torque production. Given the relatively short time in which these changes occurred, it can be concluded that results were directly related to treatment rather than the passage of time or secondary to reconditioning. Most strikingly, treatment results were successful with a patient

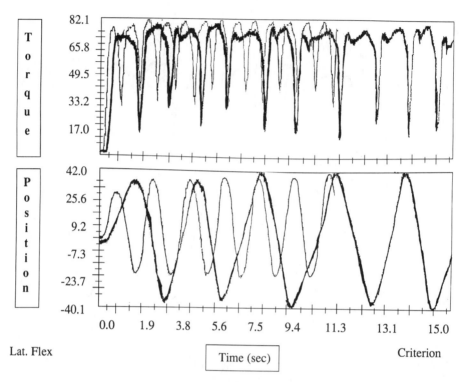

Figure 10.8 Maximum torque values produced for right and left lateral flexion; original test June 20, 1985 and follow-up test on July 17, 1985.

who had exhibited chronic back pain and dysfunction over 20 years. It must be emphasized that the test results on the Isostation B100 did not validate or diagnose the patient's chief complaint, that is, a posteriorly rotated ilium. That assessment was purely based on the clinical presupposition of pathomechanics. The treatment results, however, are validated by testing.

CASE REPORT 7: MUSCLE IMBALANCE*

History

A 47-year-old male with a diagnosis of a lumbar somatic dysfunction accompanied by paravertebral myositis was referred for rehabilitation on August 17, 1990, by an osteopathic physician. The patient was the owner and manager of a hotel and restaurant facility, but his spinal disorder resulted from his athletic pursuits as a competitive runner and road racer.

---

*By Kent E. Timm.

Before his physical therapy referral, the patient had an 8-week history of general pain in the lower lumbar spine that was exacerbated by any form of prolonged (30 minutes or greater duration) running activity. The patient's case was without a definitive mechanism for spinal injury.

Also, prior to the onset of rehabilitation, the patient had been managed by a series of osteopathic spinal adjustments which were not effective for the remediation of the patient's symptoms. The osteopathic physician theorized that a situation of general weakness of the patient's spinal musculature was responsible for the lack of success of the spinal manipulative procedures. The physician's opinion that osteopathic procedures would be more effective following a course of spinal dynamometry for paravertebral muscle strengthening was the basis for his referral of the patient for a rehabilitation program.

Evaluation

The patient presented with a principal complaint of general lower lumbar pain that delimited his athletic intentions as a runner, but that did not impose limitations on his normal occupational activities. The patient had no prior medical history of neurological involvement and demonstrated normal dermatomal, deep tendon reflex, and proprioceptive responses throughout the lumbar spinal region and in the bilateral lower extremities. The patient also demonstrated normal ranges for spinal movement ability in all three cardinal motion planes and a normal grade of strength in the T12–S2 myotomal distributions on manual muscle testing. An orthopedic physical therapy evaluation of the patient's lumbar spine revealed normal segmental mobility in all planes at each vertebral level and failed to reveal any form of vertebral positional lesion at the lumber spine or functional abnormality in the sacroiliac complexes.

Spinal dynamometry, however, yielded interesting results. The patient consented to isokinetic testing on the Cybex TEF and TORSO dynamometers, under the standardized formats listed in Table 10.1, with the spinal muscle performance results reduced for interpretation by the method which appears in Table 10.3. The patient demonstrated a normal, functional balance between the performance capabilities of his spinal rotator muscle groups, which indicated the absence of a muscle deficit in these groups but showed an unusual response for his spinal flexor and extensor muscles. Isokinetic testing revealed a 16% performance deficit in the patient's spinal extensor muscle groups accompanied by a spinal flexor muscle performance capacity that was 15% greater than the age-adjusted normal level (Table 10.3). This combination of factors represented a functional muscle performance imbalance with the spinal extensors weaker than the flexors by a total of 41%; under isokinetic conditions, extension function exceeds flexion function by a factor of at least 10% in normal subjects (16% extension deficit + 15% flexion surplus + 10% imbalance = 41%).[1-7] These findings resulted in the formulation of a physical therapy diagnosis of a functional imbalance in the patient's spinal muscle groups, secondary to conditions of extensor weakness and greater than normal flexor performance ability.

Treatment

Treatment was initiated during the same clinical session as the initial evaluation of the patient, on August 17, 1990, and consisted of cardiovascular exercise, weight training, and isokinetic exercise activities. Cardiovascular exercise was designed primarily as a warm-up activity prior to the other facets of the clinical program, since the patient already possessed a high level of aerobic conditioning, and consisted of bicycle ergometry for a period of 10 minutes at a workload level of 600 kilogram-meters per minute. This was followed by weight training exercises, using isotonic machines and the DAPRE program detailed in Table 10.4, for the spinal extensor muscle groups.

Isokinetic exercise on the Cybex TEF concluded the clinical treatment program, which was undertaken by the patient on a three sessions per week basis. The training program paralleled the isokinetic velocity spectrum format (Table 10.2), but deviated slightly through the emphasis of extension over flexion. Specifically, the patient performed the typical course of flexion/extension cycles across the speeds of 30 to 150 deg/sec, but flexion movements were performed at a submaximal force output level by the patient whereas extension exercise involved a maximal volitional intensity. These procedures enhanced spinal extensor muscle performance capabilities while preserving the patient's flexor muscle strength. In essence, the patient's spinal extensor muscles were being trained to perform supernormally to form a proper functional balance with his supernormal flexor groups.

The clinical program was complemented by the patient's own training regimen. The patient was preparing for a major 10K road race and elected to continue his usual running schedule in addition to the program of spinal rehabilitation. At no time, however, did the patient report any increase in his lumbar pain from the level of intensity present at the initial evaluation.

Progress

Treatment proceeded under the three sessions per week format until a reevaluation session on September 7, 1990. The isotonic program had been progressed in reference to the patient's spinal extension performances according to the isotonic procedures of the DAPRE protocol (Table 10.4).

Isokinetic flexion continued at submaximal work intensity while isokinetic extension was progressed in output intensity at the patient's level of comfort and tolerance. A repeat of the isokinetic testing procedures revealed that the patient's spinal flexion and extension performance scores had become equal. While functional improvement was evident, since a 16% extension deficit had been reduced to 0%, a muscle imbalance still existed because isokinetic extension output would normally exceed flexion performance by a factor of 10%.[1–7]

The clinical program continued until another reevaluation session held on September 26, 1990. At that time the patient demonstrated both normal levels of spinal flexor and extensor muscle performance capabilities and a normal relationship of extension exceeding flexion by a relative factor of 10% or more on isokinetic testing. In addition, the patient reported a complete resolution of his previous lumbar symptoms. The patient successfully completed his 10K road race on September 29, 1990, without negative incident. Follow-up isokinetic tests in October, November, and December 1990 continued to demonstrate appropriate functional capacities in and a normal isokinetic balance relationship between the patient's spinal muscle groups. The complete rehabilitation program consisted of 18 sessions over a period of 41 calendar days.

References

1. Timm KE: Back injuries and rehabilitation. Baltimore, Williams and Wilkins, 1990.
2. Marras WS, Wongsam PE: Flexibility and velocity of the normal and impaired lumbar spine. Arch Phys Med Rehabil 67:213–217, 1986.
3. Mayer TG, Gatchel R: A prospective two-year study of functional restoration in industrial low back injury. J Am Med Assoc 258:1763–1767, 1987.
4. Mayer TG, Gatchel RJ, Kishino N, et al: Objective assessment of spine function following industrial injury. Spine 10:482–493, 1985.
5. Mayer TG, Smith SS, Keeley J, et al: Quantification of lumbar function, Part 2: Sagittal plane trunk strength in chronic low-back pain patients. Spine 10:765–772, 1985.
6. Mayer TG, Vanharanta H, Gatchel R, et al: Comparison of CT scan muscle measurements and isokinetic trunk strength in postoperative patients. Spine 14:33–36, 1989.
7. Smith SS, Mayer TG, Gatchel RJ, et al: Quantification of lumbar function, Part 1: Isometric and multispeed isokinetic trunk strength measures in sagittal and axial planes in normal subjects. Spine 10:757–764, 1985.

Index

McMillan, Mary, 17
Mechanic, David, 93–94
Medication
  addiction to, 118–119
  withdrawal, 118–120
MedX Lumbar Extension Machine, 210
Mennell, John, 4–5, 12, 17
Microdiscectomy, 77–78
  rehabilitation after, case study
      of, 245–248
Million Behavioral Health Inventory, 105
Minnesota Multiphasic Personality Inven-
      tory, 91–92, 105
Movement
  as guide to exercise prescription, 41–44
  patterns of
    dynamic dysfunction (morphologic),
        41–42
    static dysfunction (morphologic),
        41–42
MPQ. *See* McGill Pain Questionnaire
Multidimensional Pain Inventory, 97, 105
Multidisciplinary pain clinic, 88–89
Muscle(s). *See also* Abdominal muscles;
      Back muscles
  coordination, changes in response to
      pain, 27
  dysfunction, 154
  exertion (action)
    isoinertial, 206
    isokinetic, 206
    isometric, 206–207
    isotonic, 206
  failure, peripheral sites of, 152, 152*f*
  fatigue
    assessment, EMG methods for,
        158–173
    central, 152
    as continuous process, 151
    contractile, 152
    definition of, 149–153, 207
    electrophysiological, 152
    in low back pain, 147–179
    measurement of, 149
    metabolic, 152
    and muscle injury, 155–156
    peripheral (localized), 151–152
    sites or mechanisms of, 149
  injury
    and fatigue, 155–156
    indirect, 156
    prevention, 156
    strain, 156
  performance, 207–208

phasic, 13, 14*t*
postoperative healing, 75
rotation effect, 153–154
strain, 12
strength, 207
  definition of, 33
  measurement of, 207–208
  static (isometric), measurement of,
      208–213
  tonic, 13, 14*t*
  training, 13
Muscle energy technique, 16
Muscle imbalances, 13–15, 24
  active, 13
  case study of, 270–273
  contribution to low back pain, 34
  passive, 13
Myofascial pain syndrome, spreading of
      pain in, 102
Myofascial release, 17–18
  indications for, 26–27

Narcotics, perioperative use of, 73
Natick upright pull tests, 225
Nervous system, role in treatment, 15
Neuromuscular reeducation, 15
Neuromuscular system, in treatment,
      15–19
Neuroreflexive change, 17
Nightingale-Conant Corporation, 142
Nociception, 88
Nonsteroidal anti-inflammatory drugs, pe-
      rioperative management of, 73–74
Nutrition, preoperative management, 74

Observation, of patient, 22
Occupational history, 104
Open-mindedness, importance of, 27–28
Operant learning, 95
Orthotics, in postoperative rehabilitation,
      79–82, 81*f*
Osteopathy, 6–7
  indications for, 26
Osteoporosis, 81

Pain. *See also* Leg pain; Low back pain
  acute
    versus chronic, 90, 92
    treatment, 115
  chronic
    benign nature of, 116
    coexisting with other illness, 104
    development of, 90–91, 91*f*
    evaluation and treatment of, 88